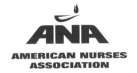

AMERICAN NURSES ASSOCIATION

D0825337

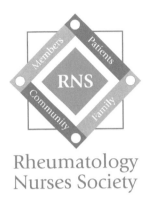

Rheumatology
Nurses Society

Scope AND
Standards
OF PRACTICE

Rheumatology Nursing

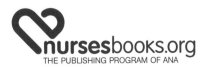

nursesbooks.org
THE PUBLISHING PROGRAM OF ANA

American Nurses Association
Silver Spring, Maryland
2013

American Nurses Association
8515 Georgia Avenue, Suite 400
Silver Spring, MD 20910-3492
1-800-274-4ANA
http://www.NursingWorld.org

Published by Nursesbooks.org
The Publishing Program of ANA
http://www.Nursesbooks.org/

The Rheumatology Nurses Society (RNS) and the American Nurses Association (ANA) are national professional associations. This joint RNS–ANA publication—*Rheumatology Nursing: Scope and Standards of Practice*—reflects the thinking of the practice specialty of rheumatology nursing on various issues and should be reviewed in conjunction with state board of nursing policies and practices. State law, rules, and regulations govern the practice of nursing, while *Rheumatology Nursing: Scope and Standards of Practice* guides rheumatology registered nurses in the application of their professional skills and responsibilities.

The Rheumatology Nurses Society is a professional organization committed to the professional development and education of nurses to benefit its members and their patients, their families, and their communities. The RNS vision is to lead nurses to excellence in the care of patients with rheumatologic diseases through preparation in the scientific basis of nursing, meeting prescribed standards of education and clinical competence, and serving as integral members of the healthcare team as patient counselors, patient educators, and patient advocates.

The American Nurses Association is the only full-service professional organization representing the interests of the nation's 3.1 million registered nurses through its constituent/state nurses associations and its organizational affiliates. The ANA advances the nursing profession by fostering high standards of nursing practice, promoting the rights of nurses in the workplace, projecting a positive and realistic view of nursing, and by lobbying the Congress and regulatory agencies on health care issues affecting nurses and the public.

ISBN-13: 978-1-55810-515-7   SAN: 851-3481   01/2014R

First printing: August 2013.
Second printing: January 2014.

Contents

Contributors   v

Introduction   1

Scope of Rheumatology Nursing Practice   **3**
  History of Rheumatoid Conditions   3
  Rheumatology Nursing Practice Environments   5
    Outpatient Settings   5
    Infusion Suites   8
    Acute Care Settings   9
    Other Settings   9
    Research Facilities   10
  Roles and Responsibilities of Rheumatology Nurses   11
  Pain Management in Rheumatology Nursing   12
  Electronic Health Records in Rheumatology Nursing   14
  Populations Served by Rheumatology Nurses   15
    Pediatric Population   15
    Adult Population   16
    Geriatric Population   18
    Summary of the Rheumatology Nursing Population   19
  Educational Preparation for Rheumatology Nursing   20
  Interprofessional Teams, Including the RN and Healthcare Consumer   24
  Trends and Issues in Rheumatology Nursing   25
    Workplace Safety   26
    Genetics   26
    Rehabilitation   27
    Ethics   27
    Advocacy   28
    ICD-10-CM   29
  Summary of the Scope of Rheumatology Nursing   29

Standards of Rheumatology Nursing Practice   33

Standards of Practice for Rheumatology Nursing   34
   Standard 1. Assessment   34
   Standard 2. Diagnosis   36
   Standard 3. Outcomes Identification   37
   Standard 4. Planning   39
   Standard 5. Implementation   42
      Standard 5A. Coordination of Care   45
      Standard 5B. Health Teaching and Health Promotion   46
      Standard 5C. Consultation   48
      Standard 5D. Prescriptive Authority and Treatment   49
   Standard 6. Evaluation   50

Standards of Professional Performance for Rheumatology Nursing   52
   Standard 7. Ethics   52
   Standard 8. Education   54
   Standard 9. Evidence-Based Practice and Research   56
   Standard 10. Quality of Practice   57
   Standard 11. Communication   59
   Standard 12. Leadership   60
   Standard 13. Collaboration   62
   Standard 14. Professional Practice Evaluation   64
   Standard 15. Resource Utilization   65
   Standard 16. Environmental Health   67

Glossary   69

References   73

Bibliography   75

Appendix A. *Outcome Standards for Rheumatology Nursing
Practice* (**1983**)   77

Index   89

Contributors

Writing Group

Deborah Hicks, RN, Chair

Ruth Busch, MSN, RN, ARNP, BC

Debra Carothers, RN

Marilyn Dougherty, MA, RN

Nicole Furfaro, MSN, ARNP

Regina Greco, MSN, RN

Joyce Kortan, RN

Betty B. Loflin, MSN, FNP-BC

Angie Tyree, RN

RNS Board Liaison

Deanna Harris, BSN, RN

Consultant

Belinda E. Puetz, PhD, RN

ANA Staff

Carol Bickford, PhD, RN-BC, CPHIMS – Content editor

Maureen E. Cones, Esq. – Legal counsel

Yvonne Daley Humes, MSA – Project coordinator

Eric Wurzbacher, BA – Project editor

About the Rheumatology Nurses Society

The Rheumatology Nurses Society (RNS) is a professional organization committed to the professional development and education of nurses to benefit its members and their patients, their families, and their communities. The RNS vision is to lead nurses to excellence in the care of patients with rheumatologic diseases through preparation in the scientific basis of nursing, meeting prescribed standards of education and clinical competence, and serving as integral members of the healthcare team as patient counselors, patient educators, and patient advocates.

About the American Nurses Association

The American Nurses Association (ANA) is the only full-service professional organization representing the interests of the nation's 3.1 million registered nurses through its constituent/state nurses associations and its organizational affiliates. The ANA advances the nursing profession by fostering high standards of nursing practice, promoting the rights of nurses in the workplace, projecting a positive and realistic view of nursing, and by lobbying the Congress and regulatory agencies on health care issues affecting nurses and the public.

About Nursesbooks.org, The Publishing Program of ANA

Nursesbooks.org publishes books on ANA core issues and programs, including ethics, leadership, quality, specialty practice, advanced practice, and the profession's enduring legacy. Best known for the foundational documents of the profession on nursing ethics, scope and standards of practice, and social policy, Nursesbooks.org is the publisher for the professional, career-oriented nurse, reaching and serving nurse educators, administrators, managers, and researchers as well as staff nurses in the course of their professional development.

Introduction

The Rheumatology Nurses Society (RNS) has demonstrated its commitment to serve healthcare consumers and their families by developing *Rheumatology Nursing: Scope and Standards of Practice*. This publication defines the scope of practice and educational requirements for nurses in the specialty of rheumatology nursing. The autonomy, accountability, and responsibilities of the rheumatology registered nurse are defined in this document.

Rheumatology registered nurses have a strong knowledge of the immune system and how it relates to rheumatic diseases. The rheumatology registered nurse has knowledge of autoimmune and inflammatory diseases, including but not limited to psoriatic arthritis and psoriasis, rheumatoid arthritis, systemic lupus erythematosus (SLE), fibromyalgia, ankylosing spondylitis and the spondyloarthropathies, scleroderma, iritis, and multiple forms of vasculitis (Klippel, Stone, Crofford, & White, 2008).

The rheumatology registered nurse understands the complex medications and protocols used to treat autoimmune diseases such as disease-modifying antirheumatic drugs (DMARDs) including antimalarials, nonsteroidal anti-inflammatory drugs (NSAIDs), biologics (American College of Rheumatology [ACR], 2010a), narcotic and nonnarcotic pain medications, and steroids. The rheumatology nurse is familiar with the use of multiple drug combinations and protocols to treat rheumatic diseases, the expected outcomes, the side-effect profiles and monitoring measures, and the interactions with other prescribed medications and nutraceuticals. The rheumatology registered nurse educates the healthcare consumer about the safe use of these agents, the need for monitoring and observation, and the need for regimen modification (e.g., withholding medications while treating a concurrent infection, adjusting doses pre- and post-op, dealing with live virus vaccine concerns), as well as the healthcare consumer's responsibility to inform all healthcare providers of all medications. Some of the medications used to treat rheumatic conditions are given in a healthcare setting. The administration of infusible medications requires the expertise of a rheumatology registered nurse with competencies in intravenous infusion technique, specific drug infusion criteria, and management of adverse and serious infusion reactions. The rheumatology registered nurse is able to take appropriate action regarding adverse events, as well as to identify insufficient therapeutic effects. The rheumatology registered nurse communicates these events to the prescribing provider.

The diagnosis of rheumatic disease requires not only a comprehensive personal and family medical history, but also a careful interview relating to sometimes subtle symptomatology. In addition, laboratory, radiographic, and other studies may be necessary to complete the diagnosis. The rheumatology registered nurse coordinates those studies with other providers and assists and communicates with the healthcare consumer and family during the process (ACR, n.d.; American Nurses Association [ANA], 2010).

The advanced practice registered nurse (APRN) in rheumatology performs physical exams and recognizes signs and symptoms of rheumatic disease. The APRN orders appropriate lab and other tests, makes diagnoses, and prescribes treatment plans. The APRN in rheumatology follows the healthcare consumer throughout the treatment program.

The Standards of Rheumatology Nursing Practice define the criteria relative to nursing accountability in the delivery of care to the healthcare consumer with a rheumatic condition. These standards provide a framework for nurses to use in evaluating outcomes and goals of therapy. The competencies that accompany each standard are written as measurable statements addressing compliance with the corresponding standard. Because these competencies provide a means of evaluating the quality of nursing care and competency of the rheumatology registered nurse delivering the care, they can be used as a method of performance appraisal. The rheumatology registered nurse will be accountable for adherence to the current Standards of Rheumatology Nursing Practice regardless of practice setting.

The goals of *Rheumatology Nursing: Scope and Standards of Practice* are to protect and preserve the healthcare consumer's right to quality care and to protect the nurse who is administering the care. *Rheumatology Nursing: Scope and Standards of Practice* will assist in developing policies and procedures in all practices and settings involved in the care of the healthcare consumer with a rheumatic condition and the consumer's family. *Rheumatology Nursing: Scope and Standards of Practice* should also be used in the orientation of new nurses entering the specialty and the lifelong education of nurses practicing in the rheumatology nursing specialty.

Scope of Rheumatology Nursing Practice

Rheumatology nursing is the specialty practice devoted to the comprehensive care of children and adults with rheumatic conditions.

History of Rheumatoid Conditions

Rheumatology is the study of, diagnosis of, and treatment of rheumatic, immune-mediated, musculoskeletal diseases, including, but not limited to, rheumatoid arthritis, psoriatic arthritis, the spondylarthropathies, systemic lupus erythematosus, vasculitis, osteoporosis, osteoarthritis, and gout. These diseases are painful, chronic, and disabling; some are life-threatening. Rheumatic conditions have plagued humans for eons.

Ankle arthritis was noted in dinosaurs as early as 85 million years ago; in humans, arthritis was the most common ailment in prehistoric peoples, perhaps because of injury or use. The remains of Ötzi (the Iceman), circa 3000 BC, on the border of Italy and Austria, revealed osteoarthritis, as well as the possibility of the use of medicinal herbs as evidenced by the pouch of herbs discovered with the body.

Skeletal remains of North American natives and Egyptian mummies also indicated the existence of arthritis during a similar time frame. In 500 BC, willow bark became known for its ability to relieve pain. It contained a naturally occurring compound called *salicin*. Salicin was scientifically studied in the 1820s and later became known as acetylsalicylic acid. Unfortunately, it was "poisonous" to the stomach and thus very difficult to tolerate. In 1897, Felix Hoffman, an employee of the Bayer Company, learned how to isolate the compound and to minimize the gastric intolerance in an effort to help his father, who had arthritis. In 1899, acetylsalicylic acid was trademarked as aspirin.

In the 1890s, European physicians applied quinine to lesions caused by lupus, with significant improvement. In the 1940s, soldiers in the tropics taking cloroquine noted a decrease in arthritis symptoms.

Many historically relevant individuals were noted to have arthritic conditions, including Benjamin Franklin, who had gout; and Auguste Renoir, who had severe rheumatoid arthritis. These and other references to arthritic conditions have been described as far back as 400 BC, although rheumatoid arthritis (RA) was not definitively identified until the 20th century.

In the 1950s, steroids became popular for the resolution of symptoms—until the long-term consequences became evident. Although still used today, steroids are used with much more caution and with the goal of minimal to nonuse. Gold salt treatments showed some evidence of remittance of disease symptoms, but again the long-term toxicity made them a "temporary" treatment. The traditional DMARDs are still used today, often in combination and/or with biologic response modifiers (BRMs or biologics).

More recently, advances in treatment as well as early identification have enhanced healthcare providers' ability to care for healthcare consumers with rheumatic conditions. Indeed, recent changes include treating to target (T2T) or remission as a goal to improve quality of life, to extend life expectancy, and to prevent disability. To those ends, nurses have become instrumental in making diagnoses, providing education, dealing with multiple disease states and their respective treatments, and managing psychosocial issues of healthcare consumers and their families dealing with rheumatic conditions.

Taken as a whole, the field of rheumatology nursing is set for exponential growth in the coming years. Rheumatology registered nurses are involved in an exciting field that combines both science and technology with nursing care of the individual and family. With 1% of the world population having rheumatoid arthritis, and a higher percentage having another rheumatic condition, nurses must have knowledge, critical thinking skills, the ability to understand multiple rheumatic conditions with underlying diseases, and the ability to make judgments based on scientific evidence that is constantly evolving.

Rheumatology nursing is complex. Healthcare consumers with rheumatic conditions have chronic and potentially disabling diseases that affect all aspects of their lives. A chronic rheumatic disease can make pregnancy complicated and can also make it difficult for a mother to care for a child, for adults to be financially independent, and for couples to engage in sexual activity. The healthcare consumer may not be able to drive safely. The healthcare consumer with a rheumatic condition experiences a variety of challenges in activities of daily living, as well as facing the psychological and financial effects of a chronic deforming and disabling disease. Without recognition and appropriate treatment, these healthcare consumers may develop deformities leading to disability and early morbidity and mortality. The comorbid diseases that can develop (e.g., heart disease, lung disease, anemia, increased risk of infection, and cancer) only add to the difficult social and financial burdens that affect these healthcare consumers and their families.

Rheumatology Nursing Practice Environments

Nurses care for rheumatology healthcare consumers in outpatient settings such as clinics, private practice, infusion centers, acute care facilities, research facilities, home health, and other settings. In the past, individuals with rheumatic conditions were treated in acute care settings. Because of new treatment modalities, these individuals now tend to be treated in outpatient settings.

OUTPATIENT SETTINGS

In outpatient facilities (clinics and private practice), the rheumatology registered nurse:

- Conducts physical assessments that are rheumatology-centric, which may include gait observations; joint counts; skin assessments; joint mobility assessments; assessments for comorbid conditions, such as infection and concurrent illnesses; lung function/breath sounds; and cardiac rhythm.

- Teaches healthcare consumers and their families about the rheumatic condition and treatment options, including risks and benefits of treatment vs. nontreatment, comorbidities, smoking cessation, and reproductive concerns.

- Teaches about and demonstrates self-administered DMARDs, BRMs, and self-administered anti-osteoporosis drugs.

- Monitors for side effects, including infections, drug–drug interactions, lab values, side-effect profiles, and adherence/persistence.

- Guides the healthcare consumer and family through a maze of insurance choices and financial assistance options, including pharma-sponsored copay assistance, Medicare Part B and D options, disease-specific foundations, local organizations, and low-income assistance programs.

- Coordinates care with other healthcare providers, such as making referrals to pain management or other specialists, physical therapy, social services, psychosocial referrals, rehabilitation services, community health clinics, and long-term care facilities.

- Provides psychosocial support and assistance to the healthcare consumer and family.

In the outpatient setting, the APRN uses the nursing process to manage care of the healthcare consumer with a rheumatic condition. Specifically, the APRN:

1. Assesses health status:

   - Obtains relevant health and medical history.

   - Performs a physical examination based on age and history.

   - Conducts preventive screening procedures based on age and history.

   - Identifies medical and health risks and needs.

   - Updates and records changes in health status.

2. Diagnoses:

   - Formulates the appropriate differential diagnosis based on history, physical examination, and clinical findings.

   - Identifies needs of the individual, family, or community by evaluating the collected data.

3. Develops a treatment plan:

   - Establishes priorities and devises a mutually acceptable plan of care to maximize the health potential of the individual, family, or community. This includes:

     - Ordering appropriate diagnostic tests.

     - Identifying nonpharmacologic interventions.

     - Identifying appropriate pharmacologic agents.

     - Developing a client education plan.

4. Implements the plan based on established priorities:

   - Takes actions that are:

     - Consistent with the appropriate plan of care.

     - Based on scientific principles, theoretical knowledge, and clinical expertise.

- Individual to the specific situation.

- Consistent with teaching and learning opportunities.

■ Further, the actions may include:

- Accurately conducting and interpreting diagnostic tests.

- Prescribing nonpharmacologic therapies.

- Prescribing pharmacologic agents.

- Providing relevant patient education.

- Making appropriate referrals to other health professionals and community agencies.

5. Follows up on healthcare consumer status:

- Determines the effectiveness of the plan of care through documentation of healthcare consumer care outcomes.

- Reassesses and modifies the plan as necessary to achieve medical and health goals.

6. Educates healthcare consumers:

- Provides education opportunities for the healthcare consumer and family related to health status, using additional resources when indicated.

7. Facilitates the healthcare consumer's participation in self-care:

- Promotes maintenance and restoration of health.

- Seeks and uses appropriate healthcare personnel and resources.

8. Promotes optimal health:

- Establishes a therapeutic relationship with the healthcare consumer and family to influence achievement of the healthcare consumer's optimal health potential.

9. Facilitates the healthcare consumer's entry into the healthcare system:

- Promotes available healthcare services and their appropriate use.

- Encourages appropriate follow-up care.

10. Performs the following procedures in collaboration with the supervising physician:

- Orders radiologic studies as indicated.

- Orders and/or provides any lab work or patient care as indicated.

- Performs any other procedures the APRN has been educated and trained to perform, including but not limited to specimen collection, skin lesion excision and biopsy, and aspiration and injection of joints.

11. Develops diagnostic plans and prescribes therapeutic plans in collaboration with the physician.

12. Consults with physicians and other healthcare professionals.

The APRN in rheumatology may prescribe, monitor, initiate, or alter the medication therapies used to treat healthcare consumers with rheumatic conditions, in accordance with education and management protocols as described by the APRN's respective state nurse practice act. In addition, the APRN in rheumatology can treat general medical conditions presented by the healthcare consumer. The APRN in rheumatology may also have prescriptive authority, depending on the respective state's nurse practice act or other regulatory language.

INFUSION SUITES

Rheumatology registered nurses manage rheumatology infusion suites and are directly responsible for infusing biologics and other agents for the treatment of the healthcare consumer's rheumatic disease or disorder. Many of these agents are proteins that are foreign to the individual, and thus have unique side-effect and infusion reaction profiles. Some agents can cause life-threatening infusion reactions; thus, the rheumatology registered nurse in the infusion center is prepared for these rare but potentially devastating reactions.

The rheumatology registered nurse in the infusion suite:

- Demonstrates competency in intravenous infusion techniques.

- Partners in the development of healthcare consumer-centric infusion suite protocols, including medication-specific administration protocols that include pretreatment procedures and medications and follow-up intervals.

- Assesses the healthcare consumer prior to infusions for contraindications such as infection, unexplained rash, hypo- or hypertension, change in health status, or newly diagnosed conditions that might affect administration of the prescribed agent. The nurse refers the healthcare consumer to the healthcare provider, if appropriate.

- Demonstrates knowledge of high-risk medications and other infusible medications used for the treatment of rheumatic conditions, such as biologic response modifiers, bisphosphonates, corticosteroids, and cytotoxic agents. The rheumatology registered nurse is knowledgeable regarding expected outcomes of these medications, side-effect profiles, and infusion management protocols for each medication.

- Demonstrates competency in dose calculations for weight-based medication dosing.

- Recognizes and manages infusion reactions, including the early, subtle signs of antibody reactions; and takes appropriate actions to preclude a more serious infusion reaction.

The rheumatology registered nurse in the infusion suite also may manage medication and equipment inventory, and may provide expert advice regarding vendor reliability, equipment safety, and equipment preference.

Additionally, the rheumatology registered nurse is available during infusions for conversations with healthcare consumers regarding the risks and benefits of the treatment(s), disease risks, other medicine updates, healthy lifestyle changes, nutritional information, financial information, and other similar topics.

ACUTE CARE SETTINGS

In acute care settings, the rheumatology registered nurse often acts in the role of consultant to other nurses and healthcare professionals regarding the underlying rheumatic condition. The rheumatology registered nurse is called on to assist in making the correct clinical decisions regarding use of medications, addressing concerns about exacerbation of rheumatic conditions and its impact on the acute problem, and identifying strategies that will benefit the healthcare consumer in rehabilitation, if warranted, and in post-hospital care.

OTHER SETTINGS

In the rehabilitation setting, long-term care, home health, hospice, and palliative care, the rheumatology registered nurse focuses on the effectiveness of the plan of care established by the healthcare providers. The rheumatology registered nurse notifies the provider when plans should be changed to achieve therapeutic effectiveness and meet medical and health goals.

In the faith community and schools, the rheumatology registered nurse acts as a resource for information; serves as an educator; and provides written materials for individuals, families, school nurses, and teachers who are seeking to increase their knowledge of rheumatologic conditions, enabling them to assist those in their care.

RESEARCH FACILITIES

In research facilities, the rheumatology registered nurse provides care involving medication and treatment trials or serves as a trial coordinator responsible for the administrative aspects of clinical trials. APRNs in rheumatology serve as principal investigators for clinical trials in some states, depending on the respective state's regulatory language.

Specifically related to clinical trials, the rheumatology registered nurse identifies the healthcare consumer who would be appropriate for the study based on diagnosis and ability to fulfill study requirements (e.g., understanding and completing paperwork, being consistent with lab requirements, being able to answer questions posed by the research coordinator).

The rheumatology registered nurse explains the study to the healthcare consumer. The explanation includes:

- The impact, if any, on healthcare consumer care.

- The frequency of office visits, lab tests, and forms to complete.

- Whether the study would require a change of medications.

- Whether the study would involve a placebo.

- The goal of the study, especially how the study will help healthcare consumers in the future, and also whether the healthcare consumer will benefit.

The rheumatology registered nurse explains confidentiality as it relates to the healthcare consumer's involvement in the study, with particular concern for exactly how the healthcare consumer's identity is protected. The rheumatology registered nurse stresses the fact that the essence of confidentiality is protection of the healthcare consumer's identity while the health information is shared.

The rheumatology registered nurse explains the length of time the study lasts and whether the healthcare consumer can opt out of the study before completion of the study.

The rheumatology registered nurse answers concerns of the healthcare consumer related to the study before the healthcare consumer signs the consent form. If the rheumatology registered nurse is unable to answer any question, the research coordinator and/or the physician is enlisted to speak with the healthcare consumer.

The rheumatology registered nurse provides the principal investigator with the study paperwork when the enrolled healthcare consumer is seen at the appropriate intervals. The rheumatology registered nurse also provides the healthcare consumer with paperwork at the appropriate intervals.

The rheumatology registered nurse explains how to complete the study questionnaire and reviews the questionnaire each time the healthcare consumer completes one, so that there are no inaccuracies, and to be certain that no questions have been missed.

Along with the research coordinator, the rheumatology registered nurse explains to the healthcare consumer how the periodic blood tests, if any, relate to the study. The blood test may measure the healthcare consumer's response to a rheumatology medication, or the blood test may be necessary to gauge whether the study drug is having a possible adverse effect.

Regardless of setting, the APRN in rheumatology conducts or participates in research according to the Code of Federal Regulations (known as the CFR Codes) and the Good Clinical Practice: Consolidated Guidelines (ICH-E6) International Conference on Harmonization (known as the ICH-GCP Guidelines). These are the "gold standard" guidelines in research.

Roles and Responsibilities of Rheumatology Nurses

Regardless of practice area, the rheumatology registered nurse advocates for the healthcare consumer to whom care is being provided. The rheumatology registered nurse is often responsible for coordinating new therapies and reimbursement with insurance companies. The laws, regulations, and policies related to coverage and reimbursement are often complex, and the nurse must have the knowledge to approach these operational challenges. The rheumatology registered nurse is responsible for counseling the healthcare consumer about coverage and reimbursement issues with new therapies, as well as navigating disability determinations. The rheumatology registered nurse will assist other providers with issues related to short- and long-term disability, and with Family and Medical Leave Act concerns.

The rheumatology registered nurse uses evidence-based nursing knowledge in the implementation of nursing care activities in practice settings. For example, the rheumatology registered nurse knows that infection is a primary concern for the healthcare consumer with a rheumatic condition. The healthcare consumer who takes steroids is more at risk for infection than an individual who is taking DMARDs or BRMs. Rheumatology registered nurses use evidence-based practice in consulting with staff on the acute care unit on which the healthcare consumer is housed following surgery. They advise about reassessment of the use of the DMARD while the healthcare consumer is recovering from surgery. Stopping a DMARD postoperatively could lead to exacerbation of rheumatic symptoms, prolonging postoperative recovery and making rehabilitation more difficult; stopping these drugs may not be necessary in all cases.

In all healthcare settings, rheumatology registered nurses synthesize information found in published research reports, anecdotal evidence, and clinical experience to improve outcomes specific to problems experienced in the healthcare consumer with a rheumatic condition. The current paucity of rheumatology-specific studies in nursing not only creates a critical need for quality research specific to populations with rheumatic disease, but also requires that the rheumatology registered nurse synthesize data from other specialties (e.g., pain management, chronic disease) and use clinical judgment to incorporate those research findings into rheumatology-based clinical practice.

The rheumatology registered nurse is instrumental in initiating changes in nursing practice based on current research findings, and involves other healthcare providers in the process when appropriate. Further, the rheumatology registered nurse participates in the conduct of research that may influence evidence-based practice, as appropriate, based on the nurse's educational level and position in the practice setting.

Pain Management in Rheumatology Nursing

Pain is the most common reason why healthcare consumers with rheumatic conditions seek medical advice. Pain can interfere with healthcare consumers' lives, disrupting their daily activities and having a profound effect on their psychosocial well-being. Thus, the entire family unit may be affected by the pain level of the person with a rheumatic condition. Pharmacologic as well as nonpharmacologic therapies (e.g., physical therapy, exercise programs, acupuncture) are used in pain management. Even so, healthcare consumers are often left with unrelieved pain. The rheumatology nurse plays a vital role in assessing, defining, and managing pain for the healthcare consumer with a rheumatic condition.

Competencies for the rheumatology nurse in addressing pain issues include:

- Knowledge regarding disease states and the principles surrounding the pathophysiology of pain.

- The ability to identify and manage the healthcare consumer's complaints of fatigue, stiffness, limited mobility, and discomfort levels.

- Acknowledgment of how the healthcare consumer's coping skills, psychosocial aspects, ethnocultural influences, family dynamics, self-management skills, and self-awareness can affect the success of a pain management program.

- The ability to collaborate with other disciplines in an effort to effectively manage the healthcare consumer's pain.

Using the nursing process, the rheumatology registered nurse assesses, evaluates, develops, and then implements a pain management plan that focuses on the effectiveness of both pharmacologic and nonpharmacologic therapies.

The rheumatology registered nurse evaluates the healthcare consumer by identifying the symptoms and functional disabilities that the healthcare consumer experiences. Factors such as sleep, energy conservation, nutrition, physical function, and interpersonal relationships are assessed and addressed with the healthcare consumer. The rheumatology registered nurse assesses the healthcare consumer through physical examination and by using functional measurement tools effective in capturing the healthcare consumer's pain level and perception of pain. The evaluation of medication effectiveness is obtained and documented along with pain medication use patterns. The rheumatology registered nurse assesses for the possible presence of pain medication tolerance, dependency, or adverse reactions.

The rheumatology registered nurse develops a nursing plan that identifies specific healthcare consumer needs to manage both acute and chronic pain issues effectively. This includes demonstrating an understanding of both pharmacologic and nonpharmacologic modalities. The rheumatology registered nurse develops a screening protocol using laboratory parameters, pain assessment tools, and pain medication use to monitor the healthcare consumer's response to medications. The treatment plan includes collaboration with other healthcare providers and agencies that are essential in implementation of the pain management plan.

The rheumatology registered nurse interprets functional assessment tools, teaches self-care, counsels the healthcare consumer and family, and recognizes deviation from the norm along with the need for additional or different pain management therapies. Implementation of an effective pain management plan involves providing the healthcare consumer with access to community services that may positively affect the healthcare consumer's physical, psychosocial, spiritual, and economic needs. The rheumatology registered nurse assesses healthcare consumer outcomes regarding effective pain management.

The rheumatology nurse assesses the healthcare consumer and family regarding educational needs. These learning needs are developed into an educational plan that encompasses the healthcare consumer's physical and psychosocial needs. The rheumatology registered nurse then educates the healthcare consumer and family about the risks and benefits of pain medications, possible adverse reactions to medications, and effectiveness of therapies, stress management, coping skills, and problem-solving techniques.

Depending on state regulations, the graduate-level-prepared specialty nurse and the APRN in rheumatology assess the need for prescriptive and nonprescriptive pain therapies and prescribe the appropriate therapy. Referrals for collaborative care are recommended and prescribed.

Electronic Health Records in Rheumatology Nursing

The use of electronic health records (EHRs) is becoming more widespread in the healthcare environment. The rheumatology registered nurse now faces additional responsibilities in using these systems. Although each institution delineates the duties of the rheumatology registered nurse, a generalized acknowledgment of the integration of EHRs into rheumatology practice is of utmost importance.

The rheumatology registered nurse reviews EHRs for the purposes of maintaining the health status of the healthcare consumer; monitoring for and aiding in prevention of certain disease states; and quickly identifying healthcare consumers with specific diagnoses, such as rheumatic diseases, or those who have been exposed to specific medications.

The approval of certain therapies, including medications, is subject to pre-certification and prior approval by payers. To provide accurate information in a succinct manner for this purpose, the rheumatology registered nurse may rely on access to an EHR.

Polypharmacy involves definite risks to the healthcare consumer with a rheumatic condition. The rheumatology registered nurse checks for medication interactions through documentation of medication administration in the EHR.

Immediate access to medical records improves intra-institutional communication and streamlines functions in the healthcare environment. Thus, documentation by the rheumatology registered nurse contributes to the healthcare consumer's health and well-being.

The rheumatology nurse serves as an advocate for healthcare consumers. In doing so, it is essential that the nurse provide education related to the disease state and medications. Electronic references provide a valuable resource for the rheumatology registered nurse.

Although the use of EHRs has benefits in the healthcare community, the privacy of health records must be addressed. Rheumatology registered nurses observe privacy rights by not disclosing healthcare consumers' medical or personal information, by avoiding access to records without proper cause, and by not sharing personal passwords or codes.

Populations Served by Rheumatology Nurses

PEDIATRIC POPULATION

Rheumatology registered nurses who work with children and adolescents must have additional educational preparation in pediatric nursing and demonstrate competence in the care of children and adolescents. Rheumatology registered nurses who work with this population must be sensitive to the unique needs of children and adolescents. Age and level of maturity have a direct effect on a child's ability to cope with a health condition. In addition to providing safe care, the rheumatology registered nurse must educate the child or adolescent, family, and significant others about the specific condition, possible therapies (including potential risks and benefits), and any restrictions that might be necessary during therapy.

The rheumatology registered nurse recognizes that a parent's first thought is to protect the child. Parents are encouraged to permit their children to grow up as normally as possible and at the same time not allow them to take unnecessary risks. Parents are also encouraged to allow age-appropriate participation in treatment decisions, allowing the child or adolescent to grow toward independent decision-making capability while acknowledging that the ultimate treatment decisions are the domain of the parents.

Rheumatology registered nurses recognize the impact of illness on children. The child or adolescent may rebel at lab and X-ray tests and the need to take medication on a regular basis. Self-esteem may be affected, and depression sometimes occurs as these children are recognized as being "different" from their peers. Other children may appear to be doing well yet have many questions and concerns about their future. For some children, the rheumatology registered nurse may recommend a referral for counseling.

In treating children, especially teens, with a rheumatic condition, the rheumatology registered nurse addresses reproductive health concerns, including contraception, as most medications used to treat rheumatic conditions are teratogenic to the fetus. Also, various medications can render the child sterile.

With respect to all children, the rheumatology registered nurse listens to their concerns and educates the children regarding the importance of adhering to their healthcare regimens so that they may achieve their goals in life.

ADULT POPULATION

The "baby boomers"—the generation of those born after World War II—have begun to enter the Medicare system, and their ranks will swell over the next decade. This will place an enormous burden on the healthcare system as the largest ever aged population. The advent of better treatment regimens for many diseases, including rheumatologic conditions, has increased life expectancy.

The rheumatology registered nurse and the APRN will be challenged to try to prevent the consequences of osteoporosis and other rheumatologic conditions, while helping individuals deal with some of the consequences of aging. Comorbidities such as dementia and Alzheimer's, cancer, cardiovascular events such as stroke and heart failure, and the caregiver role of the families of individuals with these conditions will challenge resources and nurses' skills. It will be incumbent upon nurses to provide education about prevention, early diagnosis, and treatment options, and to advocate for these individuals as well as for this generation as a whole.

Some rheumatologic conditions, such as polymyalgia rheumatica and osteoporosis, are more prevalent in the older adult population. Osteoporosis is a major health risk for individuals with rheumatic conditions because of underlying inflammatory disease, the use of steroids, limited physical activity, comorbidities, and poor nutritional habits.

It is very common for healthcare consumers with long-term medical problems to be concerned about their health when considering pregnancy. For women with early rheumatoid arthritis or those with active disease, pregnancy should be postponed until remission or substantial improvement in disease activity. Once stable, the healthcare consumer can change to compatible medications during pregnancy. However, healthcare consumers should discuss their desire to become pregnant with the rheumatologist, the rheumatology registered nurse, and the obstetrical care provider before trying to become pregnant. Women with rheumatoid arthritis may often have an improvement in symptoms of pain and fatigue during pregnancy, but then experience worsening symptoms after delivery. As many as half of pregnant women will require some form of drug therapy to control rheumatoid arthritis symptoms during pregnancy. Recently, an expert panel developed an algorithm for the management of healthcare consumers with rheumatic conditions who are interested in becoming pregnant (Bermis, Furst, Stiehm, & Lockwood, 2011). Those healthcare consumers with stable or mild-to-moderate disease activity will need adjustments in therapy, changing from medications that are incompatible with pregnancy to compatible medications.

The rheumatology registered nurse assists the healthcare consumer in understanding the medication categories established by the federal Food and Drug Administration (FDA). Because some medications used in the treatment of rheumatic conditions can be harmful to the fetus, the rheumatology registered nurse provides contraceptive counseling. The benefit of any medication must be balanced with the potential risk. The decision about which medications to use will depend on the healthcare consumer's response to treatment, the disease activity, health status, and other individual factors. Some medications may be safe during pregnancy, but some medications have not been studied, so the effects on the fetus are not always known or clear. Women with rheumatoid conditions do become pregnant and they do successfully give birth to healthy children.

Although rheumatic conditions are commonly associated with the older adult population, people of all ages may be affected. Genes, environment, gender, age, and comorbid diseases can play a part in the development and diagnosis of a rheumatic condition.

Even though individuals may have a family history of a rheumatic condition such as rheumatoid arthritis, ankylosing spondylitis, psoriatic arthritis, or gout, having this genetic link does not predict the onset of a rheumatic disorder. For example, the HLA-B27 gene is a known marker for ankylosing spondylitis. However, fewer than 1 in 20 people (Iliades, 2011) with this marker will be diagnosed with the condition. The presence of the HLA-B27 gene does not provide a definitive diagnosis, nor does the absence preclude it. Genetic markers and family history are pieces of the diagnostic "puzzle."

Environmental and cultural factors can influence the development of a rheumatic condition and sometimes allow predictions for the course of the disease. Smoking is the major environmental factor leading to the diagnosis of rheumatoid arthritis, but infection has also been implicated as an environmental factor (Klippel et al., 2008). Repetitive movements, such as data entry or assembly line jobs, can cause joint stress leading to conditions such as osteoarthritis and carpal tunnel syndrome or the exacerbation of existing joint damage caused by rheumatoid arthritis. Obesity adds additional stress to affected joints.

The occurrence of gout has dramatically increased over the past 20 years (Goodman, 2011). This increase may reflect a greater number of risk factors, such as obesity, hypertension, and a Western dietary pattern with red meat consumption. African Americans have a higher prevalence than Caucasians, possibly because of the high incidence of hypertension among African Americans (Klippel et al., 2008). Obesity is implicated in many medical conditions and complicates the treatment of rheumatic diseases, particularly since cardiovascular disease is the major cause of death in rheumatoid arthritis (Klippel et al., 2008).

Some diseases affect one gender more than the other. Systemic lupus erythematosus (SLE) and rheumatoid arthritis affect more women than men. SLE occurs predominantly in young women during reproductive years and has a strong minority representation. Ankylosing spondylitis is commonly diagnosed in young adult males. Gout is more prevalent in men and postmenopausal women. Of individuals with fibromyalgia, 80 to 90% are women (*Fibromyalgia*, 2011).

The relationship between a rheumatic condition and other diseases creates a challenge. Each concurrent condition affects the others, so balancing the risks and benefits of all the treatment plans is complicated. Healthcare consumers with gout may be obese, hypertensive, diabetic, and have renal insufficiency. Using diuretics can exacerbate gout. These physical conditions often lead to depression, confounding treatment even more.

GERIATRIC POPULATION

The rheumatology registered nurse incorporates evidence-based nursing knowledge when caring for special populations, such as older adults. The rheumatology registered nurse involves caregivers of older adults in development of the individualized plan for the healthcare consumer, thereby helping to ensure that the healthcare consumer adheres to the plan, and educates both the healthcare consumer and the caregiver about the treatment regimen.

The rheumatology registered nurse assesses for alteration in the healthcare consumer's ability to perform activities of daily living and provides education on adaptations for both the healthcare consumer and the caregiver.

In the case of an older adult with early-stage dementia, the rheumatology registered nurse assesses the healthcare consumer's ability to comprehend the treatment plan and educates the individual and the caregiver about the plan. In addition, the rheumatology registered nurse communicates with healthcare providers with whom the healthcare consumer interacts to ensure coordinated care and avoid fragmentation. The rheumatology registered nurse educates the caregiver, for example, that medical records, test results, and medication administration records should be provided from one healthcare venue to the next, using strategies such as lists, spreadsheets, journals, calendars, and others.

The rheumatology registered nurse, recognizing the costly nature of caregiving, identifies appropriate organizational and community resources that may be accessed to provide services to address the healthcare consumer's and/or the caregiver's needs. Further, the rheumatology registered nurse works to facilitate and coordinate those services to avoid fragmentation and duplication.

An essential component in rheumatology nursing of the older adult is to ensure safety, both at home and in healthcare facilities. The rheumatology registered nurse works with both the healthcare consumer and the caregiver to ensure that safety is addressed in all aspects of the healthcare consumer's life. Further, the rheumatology registered nurse takes the lead in communicating safety plans and strategies to others involved in care of the healthcare consumer, and coordinates inclusion of additional healthcare providers (e.g., nutritionists) when appropriate and necessary.

Some older adults for whom rheumatology registered nurses care are residents of assisted living facilities or nursing homes. The rheumatology registered nurse assumes responsibility for communicating care plans to those caring for the healthcare consumer in these facilities and follows up to ensure that care is being provided as prescribed.

SUMMARY OF THE RHEUMATOLOGY NURSING POPULATION

Regardless of the age at which a healthcare consumer is diagnosed with a rheumatic condition, the effect on the person's life is significant as the individual learns to cope with a chronic health condition. Children and teens may have problems with self-image, as they are less likely to be able to participate in sports and normal physical activities. Family and personal relationships might become difficult. In addition, the family may experience a sense of loss about having a child who has a compromising health condition—one who is less than perfect. The more support the family gives the child, the better the child's adjustment to living with a chronic condition will be.

The problems seen in the younger set often hold true for young and older adults. However, there are additional factors besides being married, having a family and a job, and dealing with financial responsibilities. The young mother living with chronic pain and physical limitations will express difficulty in caring for her children and lacking the energy to do so. She might also question her acceptability as a partner because of tiring easily and having to ask for help with tasks she normally would have done alone.

Similar issues occur with those having to maintain employment, especially with healthcare consumers who are more severely impaired by the condition or those whose job is more physically demanding. Disability brings with it financial constraints that might threaten household stability. It also affects self-image, as the healthcare consumer goes through an adjustment period of being self-sufficient to being more dependent on others. Older adults who are retired and independent and then are quite adversely affected by a rheumatic condition also have to cope with a sense of loss as they turn more to family members and others to help them with everyday activities.

Regardless of whether the population served is children, adults, or older adults, rheumatology registered nurses and advanced practice registered nurses in rheumatology provide peer-to-peer education and public awareness. They are involved in legislative efforts at the state, regional, and national levels. With advances in treatment modalities, the rheumatology registered nurse must be familiar and comfortable with discussing the rheumatic condition and its treatments, not only with the healthcare consumer and family, but also with other professional colleagues.

Educational Preparation for Rheumatology Nursing

Rheumatology nursing is constantly evolving. Nursing schools provide basic knowledge of rheumatic and immune-mediated diseases. However, the rheumatology registered nurse develops competencies in the specialty primarily from peers with clinical experience and expertise. Registered nurses practicing in rheumatology have initial educational preparation at the diploma, associate degree, or baccalaureate level. All are licensed to practice by their respective state board of nursing. APRNs enter rheumatology with a master's degree at a minimum. Prescriptive authority and the scope of practice for APRNs vary from state to state based on the nurse practice act and regulatory language in that state.

The expertise of the rheumatology registered nurse stems from basic nursing education, generally followed by experience in a specialty such as medical-surgical or critical care nursing prior to entering the specialty of rheumatology nursing. Learning occurs on the job from clinical experts, including other rheumatology registered nurses, physicians, and other healthcare providers who are involved in the care of healthcare consumers with rheumatic or immune-mediated diseases. Additionally, the rheumatology registered nurse is a continuous learner, attending continuing nursing education activities; reading texts, journal articles, and specialty newsletters; and participating in other educational activities such as nursing rounds or morbidity and mortality conferences.

New graduate nurses do not generally choose rheumatology nursing upon graduation from their initial educational preparation. After obtaining some nursing experience, however, these nurses begin to view rheumatology nursing as a specialty in which they can use all of their nursing skills, because the care of healthcare consumers with rheumatic and immune-mediated diseases is complex and constantly changing. It is apparent that rheumatology registered nurses care for patients of all ages and perform a variety of activities in a single setting. In addition, the advent of biologic agents has caused rheumatology registered nurses to become more aware of the purpose and value of clinical trials and the effect of the outcomes of those clinical trials on healthcare consumers and on their practice. Nurses in rheumatology nursing are at the cutting edge of advancements in treatment of rheumatic and immune-mediated diseases.

An Institute for Medicine (IOM) report, titled *The Future of Nursing: Leading Change, Advancing Health* (2010), stated as one of its four key messages that nurses should practice to the full extent of their education and training. The IOM argued that historical, cultural, regulatory, and policy barriers limit nurses' ability to contribute to change in the healthcare system. For example, legal barriers in many states constrain APRNs from practicing to the full extent of their education. The Consensus Model for APRN Regulation, Licensure, Accreditation, Certification and Education (Advanced Practice Nursing Consensus Work Group & The National Council of State Boards of Nursing APRN Advisory Committee [APNCWG & NCSBN], 2008) was an attempt to encourage the development of consistent regulations that recognize the competence of APRNs across states. It is anticipated, given the current and projected shortage of primary care physicians, and the growth of the aged population, that the role of the APRN will gain increased significance and that legislators will become increasingly receptive to efforts to expand the APRN's scope of practice.

Rheumatology registered nurses and APRNs in rheumatology practice in settings such as outpatient venues (clinics and private practice) that permit more latitude and opportunity for independent practice than most nurses experience in acute care settings. Those rheumatology registered nurses and APRNs in rheumatology who are involved in acute care settings generally function in a consultative role to existing acute care staff; thus, they experience autonomy and independence in their practice.

Another of the key messages in the 2010 IOM report was that nurses should achieve higher levels of education and training through an improved education system that promotes seamless academic progression. Currently, there are no graduate programs that provide a major or minor focus in rheumatology nursing. Therefore, nurses are seeking advanced education in general fields such as master's degrees in nursing, as family and adult nurse practitioners, or as doctoral program graduates (PhD in nursing or Doctorate in Nursing Practice [DNP]).

Likewise, rheumatology registered nurses seek certification in areas such as medical-surgical nursing, gerontological nursing, or pediatric nursing. APRNs may seek certification in areas such as adult or family, gerontological, or pediatric nursing that complement their practice in rheumatology.

Ongoing and continuing education for nurses in the specialty occurs through peer-to-peer interactions and through educational programs provided by associations in the field of rheumatology. The American College of Rheumatology (ACR) was the first of these organizations to recognize the essential role of rheumatology registered nurses and APRNs in rheumatology (ACR, 2010b, 2010c) and provide educational opportunities.

Specialty organizations are particularly good educational resources for current scientific practice information. One of these organizations, the American Rheumatology Health Association (ARHA), was founded in 1965 (in conjunction with the Arthritis Foundation) and later became the Association of Rheumatology Health Professionals (ARHP) to support and educate nonphysician providers who care for healthcare consumers with rheumatic conditions. For example, ARHP offers a web-based program to provide education for anyone interested in rheumatic conditions. Upon completion of 19 modules, the individual receives a certificate of completion.

The American Nurses Association (ANA) published outcome standards for rheumatology nursing practice in 1983, although no specialty organization for rheumatology nurses existed at that time. In 2007, a dedicated group of nurses launched the Rheumatology Nurses Society (RNS). RNS represents both rheumatology registered nurses and advanced practice nurses in rheumatology. RNS has created educational offerings specific to the learning needs of rheumatology registered nurses, both in print and online, and continues to expand the number and type of educational materials appropriate for new and experienced rheumatology registered nurses.

In education, a curriculum is prescriptive and is based on a more general syllabus that merely specifies what topics must be understood, and to what level, to achieve a particular grade or standard. In nursing, a core curriculum describes the core knowledge that must be in a nurse's armamentarium in order to practice in a specialty. The core curriculum in a nursing specialty is used to describe actual practice in that specialty. Nursing professional development educators use core curricula for orientation and ongoing education of employees of healthcare facilities; nurses use the texts for their own professional development; employers use core curricula as the basis for job descriptions, performance appraisals, and hiring decisions. Because a core curriculum is a defining element in a specialty area, the Rheumatology Nurses Society is in the process of development and publication of *Core Curriculum for Rheumatology Nurses* Both *Rheumatology Nursing: Scope and Standards of Practice* and the RNS core curriculum project are intended to serve as a prelude to development and implementation of a certification program for rheumatology registered nurses, and, if the need exists, a specialty certification program for APRNs.

The APRN Consensus Model (APNCWG & NCSBN, 2008) delineated implementation strategies for the four types of regulation of APRNs: licensure, accreditation, certification, and education (LACE). These implementation strategies were directed toward boards of nursing, accrediting agencies, certification programs, and educational institutions. Implementation of these requirements is anticipated to occur incrementally or sequentially (depending on the recommendation) with the involvement of APRN certifiers, accreditors, public regulators, educators, and employers. A target date of 2015 was established for implementation.

APRNs in rheumatology, as well as their rheumatology registered nurse counterparts and the other members of the interprofessional healthcare team, will benefit from the implementation of the recommendations found in the APRN Consensus Model (APNCWG & NCSBN, 2008). The ultimate beneficiary, of course, will be the healthcare consumer, as a result of APRNs' being able to practice to the fullest extent of their education and training. The social contract between APRNs and society will be ensured once the recommendations in the APRN Consensus Model are implemented to ensure the safety and quality of the care APRNs provide.

The future of education in rheumatology nursing is promising. Recent advances in understanding disease pathology, genetics, and the immune system have contributed to increased public awareness of rheumatic conditions. This increased interest translates to more focus on rheumatic conditions in formal education settings such as nursing and medical programs, increased research funding for care of all aspects of rheumatic diseases, and the growth in self-help groups for healthcare consumers with rheumatic conditions and their families. Registered nurses in rheumatology are able to use basic skills taught in nursing school and expand into specialized care, both through direct patient care and through being in the forefront of education about rheumatic conditions.

Interprofessional Teams, Including the RN and Healthcare Consumer

Rheumatology registered nurses are responsive to the changing needs of both healthcare consumers and society. Therefore, rheumatology registered nurses maintain and expand their knowledge base within the theoretical and scientific domains. One of the objectives of rheumatology nursing is to achieve positive outcomes that promote health and quality of life throughout the healthcare consumer's lifespan. The rheumatology registered nurse, along with the healthcare consumer and family, share the responsibility for setting realistic goals and outcome measures. The healthcare consumer must participate in setting these goals so that this individual has a stake in the achievement of the expected outcomes. Personal responsibility should be part of the discussion when setting goals and outcomes.

Rheumatology registered nurses and advanced practice nurses in rheumatology facilitate the interprofessional and comprehensive care provided by healthcare professionals, paraprofessionals, and volunteers. Rheumatology registered nurses consult with other colleagues to inform decision-making and planning to meet the healthcare consumer's needs. Participation in interprofessional teams often reflects overlapping skills that complement other team members' expertise and create flexibility in professional practice boundaries. This team collaboration involves recognition of the expertise of others both inside and outside of the rheumatology nursing specialty. Some functions of team members may be shared with a common focus on one overall mission focused on the healthcare consumer and the family.

Rheumatology registered nurses, and particularly APRNs in rheumatology, play a pivotal role in the healthcare team. Team members rely on rheumatology registered nurses, who are generally closest to the healthcare consumer and family and spend more time with healthcare consumers, as well as being the most trusted of the healthcare professionals (Jones, 2011). Rheumatology registered nurses often take the lead in planning, implementing, and evaluating the care of the healthcare consumer with a rheumatic condition, regardless of setting.

All nursing practice is fundamentally independent practice. As with all nurses, rheumatology registered nurses are accountable for nursing judgment and actions in the course of their nursing practice. Therefore, the rheumatology registered nurse and the advanced practice nurse in rheumatology engage in lifelong learning. RNS sponsors an annual educational conference to provide opportunities for rheumatology registered nurses, both those new to the specialty and those more experienced, to obtain education related to the specialty at basic and advanced levels.

Rheumatology registered nurses are bound by a professional code of ethics (ANA, 2001) and regulate themselves as individuals through the process of peer review of practice. Peer evaluation fosters the refinement of knowledge, skills, and clinical decision-making.

Rheumatology registered nurses regularly evaluate safety, effectiveness, and cost in the planning and delivery of care. With limited healthcare resources, nurses must be cognizant of both quality and cost. Nurses must be innovative in approaches to improve access to health care, especially in regard to equitable distribution of resources (such as telehealth).

Trends and Issues in Rheumatology Nursing

The rheumatology registered nurse and the advanced practice nurse in rheumatology remain aware of trends and issues that may affect their practice. Among these are:

- Workplace safety

- Genetics

- Rehabilitation

- Ethics

- Advocacy

- ICD-10 (Centers for Medicare and Medicaid Services, 2010) coding system

WORKPLACE SAFETY

The rheumatology registered nurse supports a healthy, safe workplace. In addition to addressing physical work environment hazards, the rheumatology registered nurse and the APRN in rheumatology:

- Obtain knowledge about workplace safety, including violence and bullying.

- Understand the issues of workplace violence and bullying.

- Model healthy behaviors in the workplace, including zero tolerance for workplace violence and bullying.

- Participate in development and implementation of policies that address violence and bullying in the workplace.

- Report disruptive, disrespectful behaviors (including physical and verbal abuse and workplace assaults) to appropriate authorities.

- Uphold the nursing profession's *Code of Ethics* (ANA, 2001), which requires that the nurse, "in all professional relationships, practices with compassion and respect for the inherent dignity, worth and uniqueness of every individual" (p. 1).

GENETICS

Knowledge about genetics and autoimmune disease has expanded in recent years. Genetic factors have been identified both in the development of rheumatic diseases and in individuals' response to treatment for those rheumatic conditions. For example, research has tied HLA variability to genetic disease susceptibility, as well as immune response to therapy. About 90% of individuals with ankylosing spondylitis carry the HLA-B27 gene. This HLA gene is also associated with reactive arthritis and enteropathic polyarthropathy. One hundred genetic risk factors have been "defined" in lupus subtypes and family analysis over the past 40 years.

This growing knowledge of the role that genetics and environment play has meaning for the future role of rheumatology registered nurses. The rheumatology registered nurse will need to be able to counsel individuals about their risk for developing a rheumatic condition or passing the disease to their offspring.

Based on current and future gene and allele studies, the rheumatology registered nurse will be able to individualize treatment based on the state of the science. Competencies required for the rheumatology registered nurse in addressing genetic and environmental issues include:

- Knowledge regarding disease states and specific genetic factors that are associated with the disease.

- The ability to identify the healthcare consumer's knowledge of genetic and environmental factors and develop a plan of education accordingly.

- The ability to collaborate with other disciplines in an effort to identify genetic and environmental risk in the next generation.

- The ability to share knowledge regarding healthy and affordable dietary intake, weight management, normal BMI, and the effect of obesity on joints and inflammation.

Educating individuals about environmental health hazards (such as excess sun exposure) and instructing healthcare consumers about healthy lifestyle choices (such as nutritional health, physical activity, weight management, and smoking cessation) will continue to be an essential responsibility of the rheumatology registered nurse.

REHABILITATION

Healthcare professionals from other disciplines can assist in improving the healthcare consumer's lifestyle, such as through reconstructive surgery involving joint replacement (e.g., knees, hips, elbows, shoulders, finger and toe joints) and corrective surgeries such as carpal tunnel release, kyphoplasty, or vertebroplasty. These surgeries lead to better function and improved mobility, less pain, and enhanced ability to live independently. The rheumatology registered nurse must communicate with the surgeon, the acute care nursing staff, and the rehabilitation staff to assure appropriate holds and resumption of rheumatoid medications, likely postoperative complications specific to the healthcare consumer with a rheumatic condition, and effective rehabilitation and home care as needed.

The healthcare consumer who has been immobilized or deconditioned may require rehabilitation services. The rheumatology registered nurse is instrumental in providing guidance and consultation regarding the rehabilitation care plan. The rheumatology registered nurse's role as consultant in these instances is essential to achievement of optimal outcomes.

ETHICS

Rheumatology registered nurses and APRNs in rheumatology practice ethically according to the provisions of *Code of Ethics for Nurses with Interpretive Statements* (ANA, 2001), including those related to patients, self, and the interprofessional team as well as to the community and the profession of nursing. Specifically, ethical practice requires the rheumatology registered nurse and the APRN in rheumatology to safeguard the rights and privacy of the healthcare consumer, delegate appropriately, improve the healthcare environment, participate in the advancement of the profession, and engage in collaborative endeavors to address issues such as health promotion and health policy to improve the physical condition of healthcare consumers and their families, and to ensure a positive workplace for healthcare professionals.

Rheumatology registered nurses and APRNs in rheumatology participate in activities (e.g., ethics committees) in their healthcare settings where decisions are made that affect the healthcare consumers for whom they care. In addition, in instances where ethical concerns affect the work environment, rheumatology registered nurses and APRNs in rheumatology are obligated to ensure that ethical issues are addressed as part of the decision-making process.

ADVOCACY

Advocacy is the support and influence the rheumatology registered nurse gives to issues or causes of importance to care of patients, families, and communities and to the specialty. The rheumatology registered nurse advocates on behalf of patients, families, and communities by:

- Acquiring knowledge and competencies about rheumatic conditions.

- Understanding the medications and protocols to treat such conditions.

- Collaborating with members of the healthcare team and families in providing care to the healthcare consumer.

- Working to ensure access to care.

- Advancing the quality of care delivered.

- Adhering to the *Rheumatology Nursing Scope and Standards of Practice*.

- Upholding *Code of Ethics for Nurses with Interpretive Statements* (ANA, 2001).

The rheumatology registered nurse advocates on behalf of nursing and the specialty through:

- Acquiring knowledge about public policy that influences the care and treatment of the healthcare consumer with a rheumatic condition.

- Influencing legislative and regulatory policy related to the care and treatment of the healthcare consumer with a rheumatic condition.

- Influencing public opinion related to rheumatic diseases and care of those with such diseases.

- Working to ensure that nursing's voice is considered in decisions related to such matters as scope of practice, nurse–patient ratios, prescriptive authority, reimbursement, and safety in the workplace.

- Collaborating with associations, organizations, or groups.

ICD-10-CM

The International Statistical Classification of Diseases and Related Health Problems, 10th Revision, Clinical Modification (ICD-10-CM; NCHS, 2013), is based on the International Statistical Classification of Diseases and Related Health Problems, 10th Revision (ICD-10), a World Health Organization (WHO) classification system. ICD-10-CM is promulgated in the United States by the Centers for Medicare and Medicaid Services (CMS, 2010). This system uses unique alphanumeric codes to identify known diseases and other health problems. The purpose of the ICD-10-CM is to provide capacity to differentiate disease states, to measure care, and to improve performance in clinical arenas, among other goals.

Rheumatology registered nurses, and particularly APRNs, must be aware of this redesign of the healthcare payment system and the correct implementation of processes essential for claims reimbursement. The ICD-10-CM is due to be implemented in 2014. Ensuring appropriate and complete reimbursement for care given will ensure the best economic value for the healthcare consumer, the care provider(s), and the payers.

Summary of the Scope of Rheumatology Nursing

The history of treatment of rheumatic conditions is full of examples of unsuccessful approaches and real patient suffering. Individuals with rheumatic conditions, desperate for relief, would pursue treatments such as blood transfusions from pregnant women, sunlight therapy, exposure to radon gas emitted in caves, application of oil derived from decayed worms to the skin overlying affected joints, consumption of crow's meat mixed with alcohol, electroshock therapy, and bee stings. Now early recognition and treatment with evolving complex agents and breakthrough therapies are leading to enhanced lifestyles and improvements in life expectancy of healthcare consumers with rheumatic conditions.

This expanding knowledge will require the rheumatology registered nurses to continually update their knowledge and competencies to adapt to this new information. Rheumatology registered nurses are taking leadership roles in the management of biologic therapy, including leading organized patient education classes. The skilled rheumatology nurse educator may also address the psychological and social problems of healthcare consumers and collaborate on care with interdisciplinary providers.

Rheumatology Nursing: Scope and Standards of Practice delineates the professional responsibilities of all professional rheumatology registered nurses engaged in rheumatology nursing practice, regardless of setting. As such, it can serve as a basis for:

- Quality improvement systems.

- Development and evaluation of rheumatology nursing service delivery systems and organizational structures.

- Certification activities.

- Position descriptions and performance appraisals.

- Agency policies, procedures, and protocols.

- Educational offerings.

Healthcare consumers with rheumatic conditions require nurses who have a broad understanding of the immune system and more specific knowledge of the immune response to inflammation. The medications and other treatments for rheumatic conditions are complicated by the multi-organ nature of these diseases and the overall poor health (e.g., diabetes, obesity, heart disease, smoking, chronic lung disease) of adults and older adults with rheumatic conditions.

Additionally, these diseases affect all age groups, from infants to older adults. Caring for these healthcare consumers allows the nurse to use knowledge and skills in a variety of settings, such as outpatient care, infusion management, research, rehabilitation, and education.

The knowledge base required to provide quality care is not achieved through basic or advanced nursing education, so the rheumatology registered nurse must be a self-motivated learner with the ability to glean information from multiple sources and integrate that information into clinical practice. The rapidly expanding knowledge base in rheumatology nursing offers an exciting and challenging practice venue for nurses who are self-starters; who want to make a significant impact on nursing practice; who are challenged by the need to provide information, social assistance, and education to healthcare consumers; who are able to manage complex medication regimens; who can suggest adaptive strategies for healthcare consumers to use in their everyday lives; and who have the ability to be pioneers in a relatively new but continually evolving specialty in nursing.

Standards of Rheumatology Nursing Practice

The Standards of Rheumatology Nursing Practice are authoritative statements of the duties that all rheumatology registered nurses are expected to perform competently. The standards published herein may be used as evidence of the standard of care, with the understanding that application of the standards is context dependent. The standards are subject to change with the dynamics of the nursing profession, as new patterns of professional practice are developed and accepted by the nursing profession and the public. In addition, specific conditions and clinical circumstances may also affect the application of the standards at a given time (e.g., during a natural disaster). The standards are subject to formal, periodic review and revision.

The competencies that accompany each standard may be evidence of compliance with the corresponding standard. The list of competencies is not exhaustive. Whether a particular standard or competency applies depends upon the circumstances.

The Standards of Rheumatology Nursing Practice consist of Standards of Practice and Standards of Professional Performance. The Standards of Practice describe a competent level of rheumatology nursing care based on the nursing process. The nursing process includes the components of assessment, diagnosis, outcomes identification, planning, implementation, and evaluation, and forms the foundation of the rheumatology registered nurse's decision-making. The Standards of Professional Performance describe a competent level of behavior in the professional role.

Standards of Practice for Rheumatology Nursing

Standard 1. Assessment

The rheumatology registered nurse collects comprehensive data pertinent to the healthcare consumer's health and/or the situation.

COMPETENCIES

The rheumatology registered nurse:

- Collects comprehensive data, including but not limited to physical, functional, psychosocial, emotional, cognitive, sexual, cultural, age-related, environmental, spiritual/transpersonal, and economic assessments, in a systematic and ongoing process while honoring the uniqueness of the person.

- Inquires about family history of autoimmune disease, such as rheumatoid arthritis (RA), systemic lupus erythematosus (SLE), or osteoporosis, that may affect the diagnosis of a rheumatic condition.

- Elicits the healthcare consumer's values, preferences, expressed needs, and knowledge of the healthcare situation.

- Involves the healthcare consumer, family, and other healthcare providers as appropriate in holistic data collection.

- Identifies barriers (e.g., psychosocial, literacy, financial, cultural) to effective communication and makes appropriate adaptations.

- Recognizes that personal attitudes, values, and beliefs may affect understanding of the differences between the various types of arthritis, the chronic nature of these illnesses, and medications used to treat the condition.

- Assesses family dynamics and effect on the healthcare consumer's health and wellness, as well as the family's influence on the healthcare consumer's adherence to treatment regimens.

- Prioritizes data collection based on the healthcare consumer's immediate condition or the anticipated needs of the healthcare consumer or situation.

- Collects preliminary screening data for possible biologic medication use, such as tuberculosis testing and hepatitis screening.

- Uses appropriate evidence-based assessment techniques, instruments, and tools (e.g., Systemic Lupus Erythematosus Disease Activity Index, Bath Ankylosing Spondylitis disease activity score, Health Assessment Questionnaire) related to disease activity and physical functioning.

- Synthesizes available data, information, and knowledge relevant to the situation to identify patterns and variances.

- Applies ethical, legal, and privacy guidelines and policies to the collection, maintenance, use, and dissemination of data and information.

- Recognizes healthcare consumers as the authority on their own health by honoring their care preferences (e.g., with respect to using a biologic agent that is self-injectable vs. one that is intravenous).

- Documents relevant data in a retrievable format.

ADDITIONAL COMPETENCIES FOR THE GRADUATE-LEVEL-PREPARED RHEUMATOLOGY NURSE AND THE APRN

The graduate-level-prepared rheumatology nurse or advanced practice registered nurse:

- Initiates and interprets diagnostic tests and procedures relevant to the healthcare consumer's current status.

- Assesses the effect of interactions among individuals, family, community, and social systems on health and illness (e.g., includes the family when discussing the effect of medications on the rheumatic disease process and possible adverse reactions).

Standard 2. Diagnosis

The rheumatology registered nurse analyzes the assessment data to determine the diagnoses or the issues.

COMPETENCIES

The rheumatology registered nurse:

- Derives the diagnoses or issues from assessment data, such as laboratory data, radiological data, physical examination, and history.

- Validates the diagnoses or issues with the healthcare consumer, family, and other healthcare providers when possible and appropriate.

- Identifies actual or potential risks to the healthcare consumer's health and safety and barriers to health, which may include, but are not limited to, interpersonal, systematic, financial, or environmental circumstances, such as insurance restrictions related to reimbursement, comorbid conditions and treatments, and personal habits such as smoking.

- Uses standardized classification systems (e.g., American College of Rheumatology/The European League Against Rheumatism [EULAR] disease criteria components) for rheumatoid arthritis, systemic lupus erythematosus, and other rheumatic disease states and clinical decision support tools, when available, in identifying diagnoses.

- Documents diagnoses or issues in a manner that facilitates determination of the expected outcomes and plan (e.g., "Treat to Target" goal).

ADDITIONAL COMPETENCIES FOR THE GRADUATE-LEVEL-PREPARED RHEUMATOLOGY NURSE AND THE APRN

The graduate-level-prepared rheumatology nurse or advanced practice registered nurse:

- Systematically compares and contrasts clinical findings with normal and abnormal variations and developmental events in formulating a differential diagnosis, such as rheumatoid arthritis, osteoarthritis, or other rheumatic condition.

- Uses complex data and information obtained during interview, examination, and diagnostic processes in identifying diagnoses.

- Assists staff in developing and maintaining competence in the diagnostic process.

Standard 3. Outcomes Identification

The rheumatology registered nurse identifies expected outcomes for a plan individualized to the healthcare consumer or the situation.

COMPETENCIES

The rheumatology registered nurse:

- Involves the healthcare consumer, family, healthcare providers, and others in formulating expected outcomes that consider any physical limitations (such as decreased mobility as a result of the rheumatic condition) of the healthcare consumer when possible and appropriate.

- Derives culturally appropriate expected outcomes from the diagnoses.

- Uses clinical expertise and considers associated risks, benefits, costs, current scientific evidence, and expected trajectory of the condition (including existing and anticipated deformities and damage, such as progression of joint damage as a result of rheumatoid arthritis) when formulating expected outcomes.

- Defines expected outcomes in terms of the healthcare consumer's culture, values, and ethics.

- Includes a time estimate for the attainment of expected outcomes (e.g., it may be six weeks before the efficacy of methotrexate is noted).

- Develops expected outcomes that facilitate continuity of care.

- Modifies expected outcomes according to changes in the status of the healthcare consumer or evaluation of the situation. For example, improvement in physical activity may be the outcome for the healthcare consumer with rheumatoid arthritis as a response to biologic therapy.

- Documents expected outcomes as measurable goals.

ADDITIONAL COMPETENCIES FOR THE GRADUATE-LEVEL-PREPARED RHEUMATOLOGY NURSE AND THE APRN

The graduate-level-prepared rheumatology nurse or advanced practice registered nurse:

- Identifies expected outcomes that incorporate scientific evidence and are achievable through implementation of evidence-based practices.

- Identifies expected outcomes that incorporate cost and clinical effectiveness, healthcare consumer satisfaction, and continuity and consistency among providers.

- Differentiates outcomes that require care process interventions from those that require system-level interventions.

Standard 4. Planning

The rheumatology registered nurse develops a plan that prescribes strategies and alternatives to attain expected outcomes.

COMPETENCIES

The rheumatology registered nurse:

- Develops an individualized plan in partnership with the healthcare consumer, family, and others considering the healthcare consumer's characteristics or situation, including but not limited to values, beliefs, spiritual and health practices, preferences, choices (e.g., lifestyle, smoking history, consumption of alcohol), developmental level, coping style, culture and environment, and available technology.

- Formulates plans that are specific to the needs of the healthcare consumer with a rheumatic condition (e.g., considering the mobility or pain issues of the healthcare consumer with rheumatoid arthritis, or fall prevention and exercise programs for the healthcare consumer with osteoporosis).

- Establishes priorities in the plan, such as pain control and preservation of function, with the healthcare consumer, family, and others as appropriate.

- Includes strategies in the plan to address each of the identified diagnoses or issues. These strategies may include, but are not limited to:

  - Restoring health, if possible (e.g., smoking cessation, weight reduction, diabetes control);

  - Maintaining and stabilizing health status if restoration of health is not possible;

  - Preventing illness, injury, and disease;

  - Alleviating suffering (such as when weight reduction decreases the load on weight-bearing joints); and

  - Providing supportive care for those who are dying (referral and consultation to hospice as appropriate, adequate pain relief, nutritional supplements).

■ Specifies strategies for health and wellness across the lifespan, such as encouraging tuberculin testing in healthcare consumers who are on immunosuppressant therapy.

■ Provides for continuity in the plan.

■ Incorporates an implementation pathway or timeline in the plan, such as follow-up within six weeks of starting methotrexate to assess for effectiveness and/or side effects.

■ Considers the economic impact of the plan on the healthcare consumer, family, caregivers, or other affected parties.

■ Facilitates the provision of financial assistance when needed through disease-specific foundations (e.g., Healthwell Foundation, Patient Access Network Foundation), pharmaceutical company compassionate programs, and available community resources.

■ Integrates current scientific evidence, trends, and research with alteration of the plan if new evidence emerges.

■ Uses the plan to provide direction to other members of the healthcare team.

■ Explores practice settings and safe space and time for the nurse and the healthcare consumer to explore suggested, potential, and alternative options (such as alternate sites of care, multiple medication options including generics depending on financial impact, religious objections, or other issues).

■ Defines the plan to reflect current statutes, rules and regulations, and standards.

■ Modifies the plan according to the ongoing assessment of the healthcare consumer's response and other outcome indicators.

■ Documents the plan in a manner that uses standardized language or recognized terminology.

ADDITIONAL COMPETENCIES FOR THE GRADUATE-LEVEL-PREPARED RHEUMATOLOGY NURSE AND THE APRN

The graduate-level-prepared rheumatology nurse or advanced practice registered nurse:

- Identifies assessment strategies, diagnostic strategies, and therapeutic interventions that reflect current evidence, including data, research, literature, expert clinical knowledge, and treat-to-target guidelines for healthcare consumers with rheumatoid arthritis.

- Selects or designs strategies to meet the multifaceted needs of healthcare consumers with complex rheumatic conditions.

- Includes a synthesis of the healthcare consumer's values and beliefs regarding nursing and medical therapies in the plan.

- Leads the design and development of interprofessional processes to address the identified diagnosis or issue.

- Actively participates in the development and continuous improvement of systems that support the planning process.

Standard 5. Implementation

The rheumatology registered nurse implements the identified plan.

COMPETENCIES

The rheumatology registered nurse:

- Partners with the healthcare consumer, family, significant others, and caregivers as appropriate to implement the plan in a safe, realistic, and timely manner.

- Demonstrates caring behaviors toward healthcare consumers, significant others, and groups of people receiving care.

- Uses technology to measure, record in electronic health records (EHRs), retrieve healthcare consumer data, implement the nursing process, and enhance nursing practice.

- Uses evidence-based interventions (e.g., exercise to reduce joint pain and to increase mobility, alternative/complementary approaches, stress reduction techniques proven to be effective in specific rheumatic conditions) and other treatments specific to the diagnosis or problem.

- Provides holistic care that addresses the needs of diverse populations across the lifespan.

- Advocates for health care that is sensitive to the needs of healthcare consumers, with particular emphasis on the needs of diverse populations.

- Applies appropriate knowledge of major health problems and cultural diversity in implementing the plan of care.

- Implements the plan of care by providing the healthcare consumer with education regarding rheumatology-specific medications, including the need to report the presence of possible infections; and the disease state, such as acknowledging the systemic effects of rheumatoid arthritis or the possible multisystem impact of systemic lupus erythematosus.

- Applies available healthcare technologies, such as the electronic health record (EHR), to maximize access and optimize outcomes for healthcare consumers.

- Uses community resources (e.g., state health department to address positive hepatitis test prior to initiation of biologics) and systems to implement the plan.

- Collaborates with healthcare providers, such as physical or occupational therapies, or specialty providers, such as nephrology, neurology, pulmonology, or endocrinology, to implement and integrate the plan.

- Accommodates different styles of communication used by healthcare consumers, families, and healthcare providers (e.g., uses video for visual learners, or demonstration and return demonstration on the use of self-injectable medications for learners with literacy problems).

- Integrates traditional and complementary healthcare practices as appropriate.

- Implements the plan in a timely manner in accordance with safety goals (e.g., The Joint Commission National Patient Safety Goals [NPSGs], 2010).

- Promotes the healthcare consumer's capacity for the optimal level of participation and problem-solving.

- Documents implementation and any modifications, including changes or omissions, of the identified plan.

ADDITIONAL COMPETENCIES FOR THE GRADUATE-LEVEL-PREPARED RHEUMATOLOGY NURSE AND THE APRN

The graduate-level-prepared rheumatology nurse or advanced practice registered nurse:

- Facilitates use of systems, organizations, and community resources, such as rheumatology support group meetings, to implement the plan.

- Supports collaboration with nursing and other colleagues to implement the plan.

- Incorporates new knowledge and strategies to initiate changes in nursing care practices if desired outcomes are not achieved.

- Assumes responsibility for safe and efficient implementation of the plan.

- Uses advanced communication skills to promote relationships between nurses and healthcare consumers to provide a context for open discussion of the healthcare consumer's experiences and to improve healthcare consumer outcomes, particularly in reference to adherence to the treatment regimen.

- Actively participates in the development and continuous improvement of systems that support implementation of the plan.

Standard 5A. Coordination of Care

The rheumatology registered nurse coordinates care delivery.

COMPETENCIES

The rheumatology registered nurse:

- Organizes the components of the plan.

- Manages a healthcare consumer's care so as to maximize independence and quality of life.

- Assists the healthcare consumer to identify options for alternative care.

- Communicates with the healthcare consumer, family, and system during transitions in care, such as during the rehabilitation phase following joint replacement surgery.

- Advocates for the delivery of dignified and humane care by the interprofessional team.

- Documents the coordination of care.

ADDITIONAL COMPETENCIES FOR THE GRADUATE-LEVEL-PREPARED RHEUMATOLOGY NURSE AND THE APRN

The graduate-level-prepared rheumatology nurse or advanced practice registered nurse:

- Provides leadership in the coordination of interprofessional health care, such as for physical therapy or specialty referral, for integrated delivery of care services to the healthcare consumer.

- Synthesizes data and information to prescribe necessary system and community support measures, including modifications of surroundings.

Standard 5B. Health Teaching and Health Promotion

The rheumatology registered nurse employs strategies to promote health and a safe environment.

COMPETENCIES

The rheumatology registered nurse:

- Provides health teaching that addresses such topics as healthy lifestyles, risk-reducing behaviors, developmental needs, activities of daily living, and preventive self-care (e.g., arthritis self-management programs, smoking cessation programs, arthritis water aerobics, nutritional and weight-loss programs).

- Uses health promotion and health teaching methods appropriate to the situation and the healthcare consumer's values, beliefs, health practices, developmental level, learning needs, readiness and ability to learn, language preference, spirituality, culture, and socioeconomic status.

- Seeks opportunities for feedback and evaluation (e.g., Health Assessment Questionnaire, joint counts, pain visual analog score) of the effectiveness of the strategies used.

- Uses information technologies to communicate health promotion and disease prevention information to the healthcare consumer in a variety of settings.

- Provides healthcare consumers with information about intended effects and potential adverse effects of proposed therapies (e.g., medication guidelines from packaging).

- Assists the healthcare consumer and family to understand disease states, comorbidities, available treatments, financial assistance for expensive treatments, and navigate appropriate sources of information.

- Provides information on scientifically based web sites (such as the Arthritis Foundation or National Osteoporosis Foundation), safety of web sites, and how to distinguish between evidence and testimony.

- Educates the healthcare consumer to avoid live viral vaccines while taking certain immunosuppressant medications, but encourages preventive measures such as flu vaccination.

- Prior to initiation of treatment, discusses possible areas of improvement, as well as acknowledging areas that may not improve (such as severe osteoarthritic changes in the knees or existing joint erosions).

- Educates the healthcare consumer about the role of the rheumatology registered nurse in the management of rheumatic conditions.

ADDITIONAL COMPETENCIES FOR THE GRADUATE-LEVEL-PREPARED RHEUMATOLOGY NURSE AND THE APRN

The graduate-level-prepared rheumatology nurse or advanced practice registered nurse:

- Synthesizes empirical evidence on risk behaviors (such as alcohol consumption while on methotrexate), learning theories, behavioral change theories, motivational theories, epidemiology, and other related theories and frameworks when designing health education information and programs.

- Considers comparative effectiveness research recommendations when conducting personalized health teaching and counseling.

- Designs health information and healthcare consumer education appropriate to the healthcare consumer's developmental level, learning needs, readiness to learn, and cultural values and beliefs.

- Evaluates health information resources in the area of practice for accuracy (e.g., an Internet site promoting a "miracle cure"), readability, and comprehensibility to help healthcare consumers access quality health information.

- Engages consumer alliances and advocacy groups (such as the Lupus Foundation of America or Arthritis Foundation) in health teaching and health promotion activities, as appropriate.

- Provides anticipatory guidance (such as written guidelines prior to administration of biologic agents) to individuals, families, groups, and communities to promote health and prevent or reduce the risk of health problems such as adverse reactions.

Standard 5C. Consultation

The graduate-level-prepared rheumatology nurse or advanced practice registered nurse provides consultation to influence the identified plan, enhance the abilities of others, and effect change.

COMPETENCIES FOR THE GRADUATE-LEVEL-PREPARED RHEUMATOLOGY NURSE AND THE APRN

The graduate-level-prepared rheumatology nurse or advanced practice registered nurse:

- Synthesizes clinical data, theoretical frameworks, and evidence when providing consultation.

- Facilitates the effectiveness of consultation by involving the healthcare consumer and stakeholders in decision-making and negotiating role responsibilities.

- Communicates consultation recommendations.

Standard 5D. Prescriptive Authority and Treatment

The advanced practice registered nurse in rheumatology uses prescriptive authority, procedures, referrals, treatments, and therapies in accordance with state and federal laws and regulations.

COMPETENCIES FOR THE ADVANCED PRACTICE REGISTERED NURSE
The advanced practice registered nurse:

- Prescribes evidence-based treatments, therapies, and procedures considering the healthcare consumer's comprehensive healthcare needs.

- Prescribes pharmacologic agents according to current knowledge of pharmacology and physiology.

- Prescribes specific pharmacological agents or treatments based on clinical indicators, the healthcare consumer's status and needs, and the results of diagnostic and laboratory tests.

- Evaluates therapeutic and potential adverse effects of pharmacologic and nonpharmacologic treatments.

- Provides healthcare consumers with information about intended effects, such as the length of time that may elapse before a biologic agent elicits an adequate response, and potential adverse effects of proposed prescriptive therapies.

- Provides information about costs and alternative treatments and procedures, as appropriate.

- Evaluates and incorporates complementary and alternative therapies (such as glucosamine/chondroitin for osteoarthritis, acupuncture, massage, and other therapies) into education and practice.

Standard 6. Evaluation

The rheumatology registered nurse evaluates progress toward attainment of outcomes.

COMPETENCIES

The rheumatology registered nurse:

- Conducts a systematic, ongoing, and criterion-based evaluation of the outcomes in relation to the structures and processes prescribed by the plan of care and the indicated timeline.

- Collaborates with the healthcare consumer and others involved in the care or situation in the evaluation process.

- In partnership with the healthcare consumer, evaluates the effectiveness of the planned strategies in relation to the healthcare consumer's responses and attainment of the expected outcomes.

- Uses ongoing assessment data, such as the Ankylosing Spondylitis Activity Score (ASAS) or Disease Activity Score 28 (DAS-28), to revise the diagnoses, outcomes, plan, and implementation as needed.

- Disseminates the results to the healthcare consumer, family, and others involved, in accordance with federal and state regulations.

- Participates in assessing and assuring the responsible and appropriate use of interventions so as to minimize unwarranted or unwanted treatment and healthcare consumer suffering.

- Documents the results of the evaluation.

ADDITIONAL COMPETENCIES FOR THE GRADUATE-LEVEL-PREPARED RHEUMATOLOGY NURSE AND THE APRN

The graduate-level-prepared rheumatology nurse or advanced practice registered nurse:

- Evaluates the accuracy of the diagnosis and the effectiveness of the interventions and other variables in relation to the healthcare consumer's attainment of expected outcomes.

- Synthesizes the results of the evaluation to determine the effect of the plan on healthcare consumers, families, groups, communities, and institutions.

■ Adapts the plan of care for the trajectory of treatment according to evaluation of response.

■ Uses the results of the evaluation to make or recommend process or structural changes, including policy, procedure, or protocol revision, as appropriate, particularly if the healthcare consumer does not have an adequate response to treatment.

Standards of Professional Performance for Rheumatology Nursing

Standard 7. Ethics

The rheumatology registered nurse practices ethically.

COMPETENCIES

The rheumatology registered nurse:

- Uses *Code of Ethics for Nurses with Interpretive Statements* (ANA, 2001) to guide practice.

- Delivers care in a manner that preserves and protects healthcare consumer autonomy, dignity, rights, values, and beliefs.

- Recognizes the centrality of the healthcare consumer and family as core members of any healthcare team.

- Upholds healthcare consumer confidentiality within legal and regulatory parameters.

- Assists healthcare consumers in self-determination and informed decision-making.

- Maintains a therapeutic and professional healthcare consumer–nurse relationship within appropriate professional role boundaries.

- Contributes to resolving ethical issues involving healthcare consumers, colleagues, community groups, systems, and other stakeholders.

- Takes appropriate action regarding instances of illegal, unethical, or inappropriate behavior that could endanger or jeopardize the best interests of the healthcare consumer or situation.

- Questions healthcare practice when necessary for safety and quality improvement.

- Advocates for equitable healthcare consumer care.

ADDITIONAL COMPETENCIES FOR THE GRADUATE-LEVEL-PREPARED RHEUMATOLOGY NURSE AND THE APRN

The graduate-level-prepared rheumatology nurse or advanced practice registered nurse:

- Participates in interprofessional teams that address ethical risks, benefits, and outcomes, particularly related to participation in clinical trials.

- Provides information on the risks, benefits, and outcomes of healthcare regimens, to allow informed decision-making by the healthcare consumer, including informed consent and informed refusal.

Standard 8. Education

The rheumatology registered nurse attains knowledge and competence that reflect current nursing practice.

COMPETENCIES

The rheumatology registered nurse:

- Participates in ongoing educational activities (such as those of the American College of Rheumatology, the Rheumatology Nurses Society, and others) related to appropriate knowledge bases and professional issues.

- Demonstrates a commitment to lifelong learning through self-reflection and inquiry to address learning and personal growth needs.

- Seeks experiences that reflect current practice to maintain knowledge, skills, abilities, and judgment in clinical practice or role performance.

- Acquires knowledge and skills appropriate to the role, population, specialty, setting, or situation.

- Seeks formal and independent learning experiences to develop and maintain clinical and professional skills and knowledge.

- Identifies learning needs based on nursing knowledge, the various roles the nurse may assume, and the changing needs of the population.

- Participates in formal or informal consultations to address issues in nursing practice as an application of education and a knowledge base.

- Shares educational findings, experiences, and ideas with peers.

- Contributes to a work environment conducive to the education of healthcare professionals.

- Maintains professional records that provide evidence of competence and lifelong learning.

ADDITIONAL COMPETENCIES FOR THE GRADUATE-LEVEL-PREPARED RHEUMATOLOGY NURSE AND THE APRN

The graduate-level-prepared rheumatology nurse or advanced practice registered nurse:

- Uses current healthcare research findings and other evidence to expand clinical knowledge, skills, abilities, and judgment to enhance role performance and to increase knowledge of professional issues.

Standard 9. Evidence-Based Practice and Research

The rheumatology registered nurse integrates evidence and research findings into practice.

COMPETENCIES

The rheumatology registered nurse:

- Uses current evidence-based nursing knowledge, including research findings, to guide practice.

- Incorporates evidence when initiating changes in nursing practice.

- Participates, as appropriate to educational level and position, in the formulation of evidence-based practice through research.

- Shares personal or third-party research findings with colleagues and peers.

- Serves as clinical research coordinator, subinvestigator, and/or investigator in clinical trials related to rheumatology.

- Completes components of the clinical trial/research process, such as (but not limited to) identification and recruitment of potential clinical trial subjects, participation in the clinical trial/research process, collection of informed consent from study participants, and accurate documentation of study results.

ADDITIONAL COMPETENCIES FOR THE GRADUATE-LEVEL-PREPARED RHEUMATOLOGY NURSE AND THE APRN

The graduate-level-prepared rheumatology nurse or advanced practice registered nurse:

- Contributes to nursing knowledge by conducting or synthesizing research and other evidence that discovers, examines, and evaluates current practice, knowledge, theories, criteria, and creative approaches to improve healthcare outcomes.

- Promotes a climate of research and clinical inquiry.

- Disseminates research findings through activities such as presentations, publications, consultation, and journal clubs.

Standard 10. Quality of Practice

The rheumatology registered nurse contributes to quality nursing practice.

COMPETENCIES

The rheumatology registered nurse:

- Demonstrates quality by documenting the application of the nursing process in a responsible, accountable, and ethical manner.

- Uses creativity and innovation to enhance nursing care.

- Participates in quality improvement activities, such as:

  - Identifying aspects of practice important for quality monitoring.

  - Using indicators to monitor quality, safety, and effectiveness of nursing practice.

  - Collecting data to monitor quality and effectiveness of nursing practice.

  - Analyzing quality data to identify opportunities for improving nursing practice.

  - Formulating recommendations to improve nursing practice or outcomes.

  - Implementing activities to enhance the quality of nursing practice.

  - Developing, implementing, and/or evaluating policies, procedures, and guidelines to improve the quality of practice.

  - Participating on and/or leading interprofessional teams to evaluate clinical care or health services.

  - Participating in and/or leading efforts to minimize costs and unnecessary duplication.

  - Identifying problems that occur in day-to-day work routines in order to correct process inefficiencies.*

  - Analyzing factors related to quality, safety, and effectiveness.

- Analyzing organizational systems for barriers to quality healthcare consumer outcomes.

- Implementing processes to remove or weaken barriers within organizational systems.

ADDITIONAL COMPETENCIES FOR THE GRADUATE-LEVEL-PREPARED RHEUMATOLOGY NURSE AND THE APRN

The graduate-level-prepared rheumatology nurse or advanced practice registered nurse:

- Provides leadership in the design and implementation of quality improvements.

- Designs innovations to effect change in practice and improve health outcomes.

- Evaluates the practice environment and quality of nursing care rendered in relation to existing evidence.

- Identifies opportunities for the generation and use of research and evidence.

- Obtains and maintains professional certification if available in the area of expertise.

- Uses the results of quality improvement to initiate changes in nursing practice and the healthcare delivery system.

* BHE & MONE, 2006.

Standard 11. Communication

The rheumatology registered nurse, graduate-level-prepared rheumatology nurse, or the advanced practice registered nurse communicates effectively in a variety of formats in all areas of practice.

COMPETENCIES

The rheumatology registered nurse, graduate-level-prepared rheumatology nurse, or advanced practice registered nurse:

- Assesses communication format preferences of healthcare consumers, families, and colleagues.*

- Assesses her or his communication skills in encounters with healthcare consumers, families, and colleagues.*

- Seeks continuous improvement of her or his communication and conflict resolution skills.*

- Conveys information to healthcare consumers, families, the interprofessional team, and others in communication formats that promote accuracy.

- Questions the rationale supporting care processes and decisions when they do not appear to be in the best interest of the healthcare consumer.*

- Discloses observations or concerns related to hazards and errors in care or the practice environment to the appropriate level.

- Maintains communication with other providers to minimize risks associated with transfers and transition in care delivery.

- Contributes her or his professional perspective in discussions with the interprofessional team.

* BHE & MONE, 2006.

Standard 12. Leadership

The rheumatology registered nurse demonstrates leadership in the professional practice setting and the profession.

COMPETENCIES

The rheumatology registered nurse:

- Oversees the nursing care given by others while retaining accountability for the quality of care given to the healthcare consumer.

- Abides by the vision, the associated goals, and the plan to implement and measure progress of an individual healthcare consumer or progress within the context of the healthcare organization.

- Demonstrates a commitment to continuous, lifelong learning and education for self and others.

- Mentors colleagues for the advancement of nursing practice, the profession, and quality health care.

- Treats colleagues with respect, trust, and dignity.

- Develops communication and conflict resolution skills.

- Participates in professional organizations and encourages colleagues to become active in professional organizations such as the Rheumatology Nurses Society.

- Communicates effectively with the healthcare consumer and colleagues.

- Seeks ways to advance nursing autonomy and accountability.*

- Participates in efforts to influence healthcare policy involving healthcare consumers and the profession.

ADDITIONAL COMPETENCIES FOR THE GRADUATE-LEVEL-PREPARED RHEUMATOLOGY NURSE AND THE APRN

The graduate-level-prepared rheumatology nurse or advanced practice registered nurse:

- Influences decision-making bodies to improve the professional practice environment and healthcare consumer outcomes.

- Provides direction to enhance the effectiveness of the interprofessional team.

- Promotes advanced practice nursing and role development by interpreting its role for healthcare consumers, families, and others.

- Models expert practice to interprofessional team members and healthcare consumers.

- Mentors colleagues in the acquisition of clinical knowledge, skills, abilities, and judgment.

- Serves as a preceptor for advanced practice students in rheumatology.

* BHE & MONE, 2006.

Standard 13. Collaboration

The rheumatology registered nurse collaborates with healthcare consumer, family, and others in the conduct of nursing practice.

COMPETENCIES

The rheumatology registered nurse:

- Partners with others to effect change and produce positive outcomes through the sharing of knowledge of the healthcare consumer and/or situation.

- Communicates with the healthcare consumer, family, and healthcare providers regarding healthcare consumer care and the nurse's role in the provision of that care.

- Promotes management of conflict and engagement in conflict resolution.

- Participates in building consensus or resolving conflict in the context of care.

- Applies group process and negotiation techniques with healthcare consumers and colleagues.

- Adheres to standards and applicable codes of conduct that govern behavior among peers and colleagues to create a work environment that promotes cooperation, respect, and trust.

- Cooperates in creating a documented plan that is focused on outcomes and decisions related to care and delivery of services and that reflects communication with healthcare consumers, families, and others.

- Engages in teamwork and team-building processes.

ADDITIONAL COMPETENCIES FOR THE GRADUATE-LEVEL-PREPARED RHEUMATOLOGY NURSE AND THE APRN

The graduate-level-prepared rheumatology nurse or advanced practice registered nurse:

- Partners with other disciplines to enhance healthcare consumer outcomes through interprofessional activities, such as education, consultation, management, technological development, or research opportunities.

- Invites the contribution of the healthcare consumer, family, and team members so as to achieve optimal outcomes.

- Leads in establishing, improving, and sustaining collaborative relationships to achieve safe, quality healthcare consumer care.

- Documents plan-of-care communications, rationales for plan-of-care changes, and collaborative discussions to improve healthcare consumer outcomes.

Standard 14. Professional Practice Evaluation

The rheumatology registered nurse evaluates her or his nursing practice in relation to professional practice standards and guidelines, relevant statutes, rules, and regulations.

COMPETENCIES

The rheumatology registered nurse:

- Provides age-appropriate and developmentally appropriate care in a culturally and ethnically sensitive manner.

- Engages in self-evaluation of practice on a regular basis, identifying areas of strength as well as areas in which professional growth would be beneficial.

- Obtains informal feedback regarding her or his practice from healthcare consumers, peers, professional colleagues, and others.

- Participates in peer review as appropriate.

- Takes action to achieve goals identified during the evaluation process.

- Provides evidence supporting practice decisions and actions as part of the informal and formal evaluation processes.

- Interacts with peers and colleagues to enhance her or his professional nursing practice or role performance.

- Provides peers with formal or informal constructive feedback regarding their practice or role performance.

ADDITIONAL COMPETENCIES FOR THE GRADUATE-LEVEL-PREPARED RHEUMATOLOGY NURSE AND THE APRN

The graduate-level-prepared rheumatology nurse or advanced practice registered nurse:

- Engages in a formal process seeking feedback regarding her or his practice from healthcare consumers, peers, professional colleagues, and others.

Standard 15. Resource Utilization

The rheumatology registered nurse uses appropriate resources to plan and provide nursing services that are safe, effective, and financially responsible.

COMPETENCIES

The rheumatology registered nurse:

- Assesses individual healthcare consumer care needs and resources available to achieve desired outcomes.

- Identifies healthcare consumer care needs, potential for harm, complexity of the task, and desired outcome when considering resource allocation.

- Delegates elements of care to appropriate healthcare workers in accordance with any applicable legal or policy parameters or principles.

- Identifies the evidence when evaluating resources.

- Advocates for resources, including technology, that enhance nursing practice.

- Modifies practice when necessary to promote positive interaction between healthcare consumers, care providers, and technology.

- Assists the healthcare consumer and family in identifying and securing appropriate services to address needs across the healthcare continuum.

- Assists the healthcare consumer and family in factoring costs, risks, and benefits in decisions about treatment and care.

ADDITIONAL COMPETENCIES FOR THE GRADUATE-LEVEL-PREPARED RHEUMATOLOGY NURSE AND THE APRN

The graduate-level-prepared rheumatology nurse or advanced practice registered nurse:

- Uses organizational and community resources to formulate interprofessional plans of care.

- Formulates innovative solutions for healthcare consumer care problems that use resources effectively and maintain quality.

- Designs evaluation strategies that demonstrate cost effectiveness, cost benefit, and efficiency factors associated with nursing practice.

Standard 16. Environmental Health

The rheumatology registered nurse practices in an environmentally safe and healthy manner.

COMPETENCIES

The rheumatology registered nurse:

- Attains knowledge of environmental health concepts, such as implementation of environmental health strategies.

- Promotes a practice environment that reduces environmental health risks for workers and healthcare consumers.

- Assesses the practice environment for factors that threaten health, such as sound, odor, noise, and light.

- Advocates for the judicious and appropriate use of products in health care.

- Communicates environmental health risks and exposure reduction strategies to healthcare consumers, families, colleagues, and communities.

- Uses scientific evidence to determine if a product or treatment is an environmental threat.

- Participates in strategies to promote healthy communities.

ADDITIONAL COMPETENCIES FOR THE GRADUATE-LEVEL-PREPARED RHEUMATOLOGY NURSE AND THE APRN

The graduate-level-prepared rheumatology nurse or advanced practice registered nurse:

- Creates partnerships that promote sustainable environmental health policies and conditions.

- Analyzes the impact of social, political, and economic influences on the environment and human health exposures.

- Critically evaluates the manner in which environmental health issues (such as the use of bisphosphonates and calcium supplements for bone loss) are presented by the popular media and clarifies this information for the healthcare consumer and family.

■ Advocates for implementation of environmental principles for nursing practice.

■ Supports nurses in advocating for and implementing environmental principles in nursing practice.

Glossary

Advanced practice registered nurse (APRN). A nurse who has completed an accredited graduate-level education program preparing her or him for the role of certified nurse practitioner, certified registered nurse anesthetist, certified nurse-midwife, or clinical nurse specialist; has passed a national certification examination that measures the APRN role and population-focused competencies; maintains continued competence as evidenced by recertification; and is licensed to practice as an APRN.

Biologics. Bioengineered replicas of human proteins that inhibit critical cytokines and immune cells that target specific immunologic pathways. These agents are used in the treatment of rheumatic diseases to improve signs and symptoms and significantly prevent the progression of joint damage.

Competency. An expected and measurable level of nursing performance that integrates knowledge, skills, abilities, and judgment, based on established scientific knowledge and expectations for nursing practice.

Complementary/alternative therapy. Originally identified as those therapies not traditionally taught in U.S. medical schools and not traditionally used in U.S. hospitals, although now taught in more than 40 U.S. medical schools. Examples include acupressure, acupuncture, herbal medicines, nutritional therapy, yoga, meditation, and homeopathy.

Diagnosis. A clinical judgment about a healthcare consumer's response to actual or potential health conditions or needs. The diagnosis provides the basis for determination of a plan to achieve expected outcomes. Rheumatology registered nurses use nursing and medical diagnoses depending on educational and clinical preparation and legal authority.

Disease activity indices. Validated health status instruments for use in the assessment of disease states. They can be generalized or disease/disorder specific and usually include patient/practitioner global assessments, disease characteristic assessments, and laboratory parameters. Examples used in rheumatology include ASAS (ankylosing spondylitis assessment score), HAQ (health assessment questionnaire), SLEDAI (systemic lupus erythematosus disease activity index), and DAS-28 (Disease Activity Score 28 [joint count]).

Disease-modifying antirheumatic drugs (DMARDs). Traditional drugs used to moderate the disease process and slow the progression of joint erosions and disability. The disease generally recurs with the discontinuation of these drugs. Examples of DMARDs include methotrexate, hydroxychloroquine, leflunomide, and sulfasalazine.

Evidence-based practice. A scholarly and systematic problem-solving paradigm that results in the delivery of high-quality health care.

Family. Family of origin or significant others as identified by the healthcare consumer.

Graduate-level-prepared specialty nurse. A registered nurse prepared at the master's or doctoral educational level who has advanced knowledge, skills, abilities, and judgment associated with one or more nursing specialties and is functioning in an advanced level as designated by elements of his or her position.

Healthcare consumer. The person, client, family, group, community, or population who is the focus of attention and to whom the registered nurse is providing services as sanctioned by the state regulatory bodies.

Healthcare providers. Individuals with special expertise who provide healthcare services or assistance to patients. May include nurses, physicians, psychologists, social workers, nutritionists/dietitians, and various therapists.

Immune-mediated diseases. Conditions resulting from abnormal activity of the body's immune system. Autoimmune disorders constitute a subset of immune-mediated diseases. In autoimmune conditions, the body fails to recognize itself, which allows immune responses against its own cells and tissues. Examples are systemic lupus erythematosus, diabetes mellitus, and Sjögren's syndrome.

Investigator. The primary individual responsible for all aspects of a clinical trial.

Interprofessional. Reliant on the overlapping knowledge, skills, and abilities of each professional team member. Interprofessionalism can drive synergistic effects by which outcomes are enhanced and become more comprehensive than a simple aggregation of the individual efforts of the team members.

Nursing. The protection, promotion, and optimization of health and abilities; prevention of illness and injury; alleviation of suffering through the diagnosis and treatment of human response; and advocacy in the care of individuals, families, communities, and populations.

Nursing practice. The collective professional activities of nurses; characterized by the interrelations of human responses, theory application, nursing actions, and outcomes.

Nursing process. A critical thinking model used by nurses that integrates the singular, concurrent actions of six components: assessment, diagnosis, outcomes identification, planning, implementation, and evaluation.

Registered nurse (RN). An individual registered or licensed by a state, commonwealth, territory, government, or other regulatory body to practice as a registered nurse.

Rheumatic diseases. Nonspecific term for medical problems affecting the joints and connective tissues.

Scope of Nursing Practice. A description of the *who, what, where, when, why,* and *how* of nursing practice that addresses the range of nursing practice activities common to all registered nurses. When considered in conjunction with the Standards of Professional Nursing Practice and the Code of Ethics for Nurses, comprehensively describes the competent level of nursing common to all registered nurses.

Standards. Authoritative statements defined and promoted by the profession by which the quality of practice, service, or education can be evaluated.

Standards of Professional Nursing Practice. Authoritative statements of the duties that all registered nurses, regardless of role, population, or specialty, are expected to perform competently.

Subinvestigator. An individual who reports to the primary investigator in a clinical trial. Performs tasks and assumes responsibility for aspects of the clinical trial as assigned or delegated by the investigator.

References

Advanced Practice Nursing Consensus Work Group & The National Council
of State Boards of Nursing APRN Advisory Committee [APNCWG &
NCSBN]. (2008). *Consensus model for APRN regulation: Licensure,
accreditation, certification & education.* Chicago, IL: National Council of
State Boards of Nursing. Retrieved from http://www.aacn.nche.edu
/education-resources/APRNReport.pdf

American College of Rheumatology [ACR]. (n.d.). *Standards of practice:
Professional nursing competencies in rheumatology.* Retrieved from http:
//www.rheumatology.org/practice/clinical/standards/nursestandards.asp

American College of Rheumatology [ACR]. (2010a). *Biologic treatments for
rheumatoid arthritis.* Retrieved from http://www.rheumatology.org
/practice/clinical/patients/medications/biologics.asp

American College of Rheumatology [ACR]. (2010b). *The role of the
rheumatology registered nurse in the management of rheumatic disease.
Atlanta,* GA: Author.

American College of Rheumatology [ACR]. (2010c). *The role of APN in the
management of rheumatic disease.* Atlanta, GA: Author.

American Nurses Association [ANA]. (2001). *Code of ethics for nurses with
interpretive statements.* Silver Spring, MD: Nursesbooks.org.

American Nurses Association [ANA]. (2010). *Nursing: Scope and standards
of practice* (2nd ed.). Silver Spring, MD: Nursesbooks.org.

Bermis, B., Furst, D., Stiehm, E., & Lockwood, C. (2011, October 19). *Use of
anti-inflammatory and immunosuppressive drugs in rheumatic diseases
during pregnancy and lactation: Summary and recommendations.*
Retrieved from www.uptodate.com

Board of Higher Education & Massachusetts Organization of Nurse Executives [BHE & MONE]. (2006). *Creativity and connections: Building the framework for the future of nursing education. Report from the invitational working session, March 23–24, 2006.* Burlington, MA: Massachusetts Organization of Nurse Executives. Retrieved from http://www.mass.edu /currentinit/documents/NursingCreativityAndConnections.pdf

Fibromyalgia (National Institutes of Health Publication No. 11-5326). (2011). Washington, DC: National Institute of Arthritis & Musculoskeletal and Skin Diseases (NIAMS). Retrieved from www.niams.nih.gov /Health_Info/fibromyalgia/fibromyalgia_ff.asp

Goodman, A. (2011). *Obese people get gout at younger age than non-obese.* Atlanta, GA: Arthritis Foundation. Retrieved from www.arthritistoday. org/new/obesity-gout-community152.php

Iliades, C. (2011). *What is ankylosing spondylitis?* Washington, DC: National Institute of Arthritis and Musculoskeletal and Skin Diseases (NIAMS). Retrieved from www.niams.nih.gov/Health_info/Ankylosing_Spondylitis /default.asp

Institute of Medicine. (2010). *The future of nursing: Leading change, advancing health.* Washington, DC: Author. Retrieved from http: //www.iom.edu/Reports/2010/The-Future-of-Nursing-Leading-Change-Advancing-Health.aspx

The Joint Commission. (2010). *2010 Joint Commission National Patient Safety Goals.* Retrieved from http://www.patientsafety.gov/TIPS/Docs /TIPS_JanFeb10Poster.pdf

Jones, J. M. (2011). *Record 64% rate honesty, ethics of members of Congress low. Ratings of nurses, pharmacists, and medical doctors most positive.* Retrieved from http://www.gallup.com/poll/151460/Record-Rate-Honesty-Ethics-Members-Congress-Low.aspx

Klippel, J. H., Stone, J. H., Crofford, L. J., & White, P. H. (Eds.). (2008). *Primer on the rheumatic diseases.* New York, NY: Springer.

National Center for Health Statistics (NCHS). (2013). *International statistical classification of diseases and related health problems, 10th revision, clinical modification* (ICD-10-CM; 2013 release of ICD-10-CM). Retrieved from http://www.cdc.gov/nchs/icd/icd10cm.htm#10update

Rheumatology Nursing: Scope and Standards of Practice

Bibliography

American Nurses Association [ANA]. (1983). *Outcome standards for rheumatology nursing practice.* Retrieved from http://www.ncbi.nlm.nih.gov/pubmed/6605098

Bartlett, S. J., Bingham, C. O., Maricic, M. J., Daly Iverson, M., & Ruffing, V. (Eds.). (2006). *Clinical care in the rheumatic diseases* (3rd ed.). Atlanta, GA: Association of Rheumatology Health Professionals.

Hill, J. (Ed.). (2006). *Rheumatology nursing: A creative approach* (2nd ed.). West Sussex, UK: John Wiley & Sons.

Iliades, C. (2009). *Diagnosing lupus: From start to finish.* Retrieved from www.everydayhealth.com/lupus/lupus-diagnosis-start-to-finish.aspx

Imboden, J. B., Hellman, D. B., & Stone, J. H. (2007). *Current rheumatology diagnosis and treatment* (2nd ed.). New York, NY: McGraw Hill.

Labunski, A. J. (1991). Behavioral competencies for nursing practice. *Nursing Outlook, 39*(4), 174–177.

Osteoarthritis (Information Clearing House, National Institutes of Health Publication No. 10-4617). (2010). Washington, DC: National Institutes of Arthritis & Musculoskeletal and Skin Diseases (NIAMS). Retrieved from http://www.niams.nih.gov/Health_info/Osteoarthritis/default.asp

Pigg, J. S., & Schroeder, P. M. (1984). Frequently occurring problems of patients with rheumatic diseases: The ANA outcome standards for rheumatology nursing practice. *Nursing Clinics of North America, 19*(4), 697–708.

Psoriatic Arthritis. (2012). Atlanta, GA: Arthritis Foundation. Retrieved from www.arthritis.org/disease_id=21

Ruderman, E., & Tambar, S. (2011). *Rheumatoid arthritis.* Atlanta, GA: American College of Rheumatology. Retrieved from www.rheumatology.org/practice/clinical/patients/diseases_and_conditions

Schumacher, H. R. (2011). *Gout.* Atlanta, GA: American College of Rheumatology. Retrieved from www.rheumatology.org/practice/clinical/patients/diseases_and_conditions

Weinstein, S. M. (2006). *Plumer's principles and practice of intravenous therapy* (8th ed.). Philadelphia, PA: Lippincott Williams & Wilkins.

Appendix A.

Outcome Standards for Rheumatology Nursing Practice (1983)

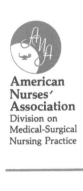

**American Nurses'
Association**
Division on
Medical-Surgical
Nursing Practice

*Outcome
Standards
for
Rheumatology
Nursing Practice*

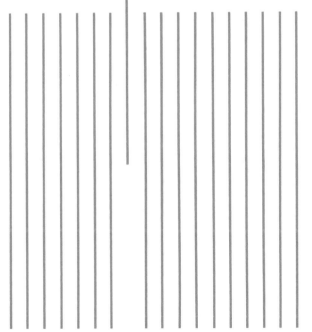

OUTCOME STANDARDS
for
Rheumatology
Nursing Practice

American Nurses' Association

Division on Medical-Surgical Nursing Practice

and

Arthritis Health Professions Association

(A Section of the Arthritis Foundation)

The content in this appendix is not current and is of historical significance only.

Arthritis Health Professions Association Nursing Standards Task Force
Marie L. Heiss, M.S., R.N., and Janice Pigg, B.S.N., R.N., Co-chair
Pamela W. Driscoll, B.S.N., R.N.
Terese M. Halfman, M.S.N., R.N.
Barbara McHugh, M.P.H., R.N.
Pat Moore, R.N.
Marita K. Murrman, M.S., R.N.
Catherine A. Novak, M.S.N., R.N.
Peggy Raish, M.S.N., R.N.
Pamela M. Schroeder, M.S.N., R.N.
Gigi S. Viellion, R.N.

American Nurses Association Division on
Medical-Surgical Nursing Practice 1980-1982 Executive Committee
Cynthia Scalzi, M.N., R.N., Chairperson
Jeanette K. Chambers, M.N., R.N., Vice Chairperson
Carol Roe, M.S.N., R.N., Secretary
Ruth Moran, Ed.D., R.N.
Margaret F. Fuhs, D.N.Sc., R.N.
Margaret J. Stafford, M.S.N., R.N.

1982-1984 Executive Committee
Jeanette K. Chambers, M.S.N., R.N., C.S., Chairperson
Laura Cross, M.S., R.N., Vice Chairperson
Carol Roe, M.S.N., R.N., C.N.A., Secretary
Lucy Feild, M.S., R.N.
Margaret F. Fuhs, D.N.Sc., R.N. (1982-1983)
Elizabeth Hahn Winslow, Ph.D., R.N.

Published by
American Nurses Association
600 Maryland Ave., SW, Suite 100W
Washington, DC 20024-2571

MS-12   3M   4/83

The content in this appendix is not current and is of historical significance only.

INTRODUCTION

The impact of rheumatic diseases on individuals, families, and society has long been underestimated. The correlation of these diseases with the aging process, the unpredictability of symptoms, and the concept of arthritis as a single disease have given rise to many misleading beliefs and folklore. These misconceptions have led individuals to delay seeking diagnosis and treatment and to regard pain and disability as inevitable. They have also led to a general lack of awareness of the economic and human costs that arise from rheumatic diseases, a serious health problem that affects over 37 million Americans.

The word arthritis is a collective term which refers to over 100 different conditions that present or have as a major component musculoskeletal symptoms such as pain, stiffness, weakness, and loss of motion. Persons of all age groups, children to adults in the prime of life, may be affected. Although primarily thought of only in terms of joint involvement, the rheumatic diseases may involve multiple body systems. Thus, these diseases, which may last the lifetime of an individual, carry with them not only the constant threat of joint damage but also systemic complications.

Because these conditions are both widespread and complex, the growing medical subspecialty of rheumatology has increasingly involved all health care disciplines, particularly nurses. The care of such patients touches all areas of nursing practice in a variety of settings. There is consequently a need for developing standards for nursing practice.

The standards offered in this document focus on patient outcomes and included rationales specific to individuals with rheumatic disease. The nursing interventions are directed towards helping the individual achieve optimal function and find personal fulfillment in spite of changes imposed by the disease.

These standards relate to the problem areas that both patients and their families encounter and are in accord with the definition of nursing given in *Nursing: A Social Policy Statement*, a document of the American Nurses' Association:

> Nursing is the diagnosis and treatment of human responses to actual or potential health problems...

These standards are also based on the following beliefs:
1. An emphasis on the individual's potential responsibility to maintain optimal health.
2. The inclusion of the individual and family in decision making.
3. A respect for the individual's right to accept or reject a therapeutic plan.
4. An emphasis on teaching self-management techniques.

It is recognized that these patient outcomes may not be effected exclusively by nurses. They are, however, patient outcomes for which the

Outcome Standard II. Alteration in Comfort: Stiffness

THE INDIVIDUAL INCORPORATES AS PART OF DAILY ACTIVITIES THOSE MEASURES NECESSARY TO MANAGE STIFFNESS.

Rationale

1. Stiffness may be generalized or localized.
2. Stiffness increases and decreases in direct proportion to the amount of inflammation present. Other factors (e.g. structural changes) may cause stiffness in a joint.
3. Overactivity, inactivity, or unaccustomed activity may increase stiffness.
4. Stiffness may be confused with or accompany pain.
5. As the intensity and duration of stiffness increases, activities of daily living may be compromised; as the intensity and duration of stiffness decreases, activities of daily living may improve.
6. The earlier the intervention to decrease morning stiffness is offered, the sooner results are achieved.
7. Anti-inflammatory and disease modifying medications may decrease stiffness.
8. Heat may decrease stiffness; conversely cold may increase stiffness.
9. Frequent changes of position may decrease stiffness.

Criteria

The individual—
1. explains the relationship between stiffness and disease activity, medication, and activities of daily living.
2. verbalizes changes in the intensity and duration of stiffness.
3. describes appropriate methods for decreasing stiffness.
4. describes a schedule of daily activities which takes into account the intensity and duration of stiffness.
5. utilizes appropriate methods for decreasing stiffness.

The content in this appendix is not current and is of historical significance only.

Outcome Standard III. Alteration in Energy Level: Fatigue

THE INDIVIDUAL INCORPORATES AS PART OF DAILY ACTIVITIES THOSE MEASURES NECESSARY TO MODIFY FATIGUE.

Rationale

1. Fatigue may be a warning of impending increase in disease activity.
2. Generalized fatigue may increase or decrease in proportion to disease activity.
3. Fatigue may be both physical and psychological in origin.
4. The severity and duration of fatigue may affect or be influenced by the individual's—
   a. degree of stress.
   b. perception of pain.
   c. sexual activity.
   d. quality of sleep.
   e. performance of daily activities.
   f. nutrition.
5. Fatigue may be associated with anemia of chronic disease or with chronic blood loss.
6. Fatigue may be lessened by—
   a. conserving energy through rest, planning, setting priorities, pacing, and assistive devices.
   b. developing effective coping strategies.
   c. controlling the disease process.
   d. using appropriate pain management measures.

Criteria

The individual—
1. explains the relationship of fatigue to disease activity.
2. differentiates between psychological and physical factors that may cause fatigue.
3. identifies measures to prevent or modify fatigue.
4. utilizes measures to prevent or modify fatigue.

The content in this appendix is not current and is of historical significance only.

Outcome Standard IV. Self-Care Deficit

THE INDIVIDUAL ACHIEVES SELF-CARE INDEPENDENTLY OR WITH THE USE OF RESOURCES.

Rationale

1. The ability to perform self-care activities is influenced by the disease activity and the accompanying pain, stiffness, fatigue, muscle weakness, loss of motion, and depression.
2. Individuals differ in their ability and willingness to perform self-care activities.
3. Individuals often make adaptations in self-care activities.
4. The degree of deformity does not necesesarily reflect the individual's ability to perform self-care activities.
5. The individual's ability to perform self-care activities independently may be influenced by the family's perception of the level of assistance needed.
6. Assistive devices may enhance self-care abilities; however, individuals react differently to the use of such equipment.
7. Changes in ability to care for self may lead to a decrease in personal safety.

Criteria

The individual—
1. identifies factors that interfere with the ability to perform self-care activities.
2. identifies alternative methods for meeting self-care needs.
3. utilizes alternative methods for meeting self-care needs.

The content in this appendix is not current and is of historical significance only.

Outcome Standard V. Knowledge Deficit Regarding Physical Mobility (Ambulation)

THE INDIVIDUAL ATTAINS AND MAINTAINS OPTIMAL FUNCTIONAL MOBILITY.

Rationale

1. An increase in disease activity may result in decreased physical activity and decreased mobility.
2. Pain, stiffness, and fatigue may temporarily limit mobility.
3. Limitation of motion in one joint places additional mechanical stress on other joints.
4. Mobility is not necessarily related to deformity.
5. The degree of mobility is not synonymous with the degree of independence.
6. Decreased mobility may influence a person's self-concept and lead to social isolation.
7. Changes in mobility may lead to a decrease in personal safety.
8. Correct posture and posititioning are necessary for maintaining optimal mobility.
9. Proper footwear and/or assistive equipment may improve mobility.
10. Therapeutic exercises may improve mobility.
11. Furniture and architectural adaptations may enhance mobility.

Criteria

The individual—
1. identifies factors which interfere with mobility.
2. describes measures to prevent loss of motion.
3. utilizes measures to prevent loss of motion.
4. utilizes appropriate techniques and/or assistive equipment to aid mobility.
5. identifies community resources available to assist in managing decreased mobility.
6. identifies environmental (home, school, work, community) barriers to optimal mobility.

The content in this appendix is not current and is of historical significance only.

Outcome Standard VI. Knowledge Deficit Regarding Self-Management Decisions

THE INDIVIDUAL AND FAMILY HAVE NECESSARY INFORMATION ABOUT THE DISEASE PROCESS AND THE THERAPY TO MAKE SELF-CARE MANAGEMENT DECISIONS.

Rationale

1. The duration of the disease is not an indicator of the individual's and family's knowledge of self-care management.
2. The individual's perception of the cause, treatment, and prognosis of the disease may need correction or clarification.
3. Factors such as pain, fatigue, and depression may interfere with the individual's readiness to learn.
4. Physical, psychological, intellectual, and social barriers may influence the individual's ability to learn and implement information.
5. The way in which information is given, not just the information itself, may influence the individual's behavior.
6. An individual may need supervised practice to incorporate self-care management techniques into daily activities.
7. The individual needs accurate information in order to discriminate between proven and unproven methods of treatment.
8. The individual may need periodic reassessment and reinforcement of what has been taught.

Criteria

The individual—
1. describes an appropriate plan for managing personal health care.
2. explains reasons for choices in personal management behaviors.
3. verbalizes sufficient information to meet self-management needs according to a personal value system.
4. identifies personal and community resources that may provide information or assistance.

The content in this appendix is not current and is of historical significance only.

Outcome Standard VII. Ineffective Coping, Individual or Family

THE INDIVIDUAL ACHIEVES A BALANCE BETWEEN THE STRESS IMPOSED BY THE RHEUMATIC DISEASE AND PERSONAL FULFILLMENT.

Rationale

1. The individual may experience stress caused by the perceived or actual nature of the rheumatic disease. Psychological and physical factors causing stress may include:
   a. fear of being crippled.
   b. fear of pain.
   c. lack of known "cause or cure."
   d. dread of dependency and disability.
   e. fear of losing significant social relationships.
   f. fear of physical changes.
   g. fear of taking prescribed medications.
   h. fear of occupational loss.
2. The exacerbations and remissions characteristic of many rheumatic diseases require continual changes in coping strategies.
3. The uncertainty and unpredictability of the disease course affects the individual's degree of control in planning and carrying out daily activities.
4. The individual's ability to cope is influenced by past experiences in adapting to change.
5. An individual's difficulty in performing self-care may represent inappropriate coping (e.g. controlling activities of others).
6. An individual's problem-solving abilities may be influenced by the chronic nature of the rheumatic disease.
7. The ability to cope is influenced by individual, family, and community resources available to meet physical, psychosocial, spiritual, vocational, and economic needs.
8. Society's misinformation about the rheumatic diseases promotes attitudes that may create stressful situations for both the individual and the family.

Criteria

The individual—
1. verbalizes psychological and physical stress factors.
2. identifies appropriate strategies for coping with personal stress.
3. revises expectations regarding amount and type of activity possible in daily life.
4. identifies available resources.
5. utilizes available resources.

The content in this appendix is not current and is of historical significance only.

Outcome Standard VIII. Disturbance in Self-Concept

THE INDIVIDUAL ACHIEVES A RECONCILIATION BETWEEN SELF-CONCEPT AND THE PHYSICAL AND PSYCHOLOGICAL CHANGES IMPOSED BY THE RHEUMATIC DISEASE.

Rationale

1. The individual's self-concept may be altered by the disease or its treatment.
2. The individual's self-concept may change because of impaired self-care ability.
3. The individual's perception of sexuality may be affected by the physical and psychological changes imposed by the rheumatic disease and its treatment.
4. The family's perception of the individual with a rheumatic disease may be altered.
5. The individual's and the family's role may need to accommodate to the remissions and exacerbations of the disease.
6. The individual's self-concept may affect self-management decisions.
7. The individual's self-concept may be inconsistent with society's attitude toward him/her.

Criteria

The individual—
1. verbalizes an awareness that changes taking place in self-concept are a normal response to rheumatic disease.
2. identifies strategies to cope with altered self-concept.

The family —
1. verbalizes role changes.
2. identifies strategies to cope with role changes.

Index

Note: Entries with [1983] indicate an entry from *Outcome Standards for Rheumatology Nursing Practice* (1983), reproduced in Appendix A. That information is not current but included for historical value only.

A

Abilities in rheumatology nursing practice, 4, 10, 46
   See also Knowledge, skills, abilities, and judgment

Accountability in rheumatology nursing practice, 1, 2
   leadership and, 60
   quality of practice and, 57
   See also Delegation

Acetylsalicylic acid, (aspirin) in arthritis, 3

Activities in rheumatology nursing practice
   challenges, 4–5
   nursing care, 11

Acute care settings in rheumatology nursing practice, 5, 9, 22

Adolescents, rheumatology nurses and, 15–16, 19

Adult population, rheumatology nurses and, 16–18, 20
   See also Population-based health care

Advanced Practice Nursing Consensus Work Group (APNCWG), 21, 23

Advanced practice registered nurses (APRNs) in rheumatology nursing practice, 2
   assessment competencies, 35
   certification, 22
   for clinical trials, 10
   collaboration competencies, 63
   communication competencies, 59
   consultation competencies, 48
   coordination of care competencies, 45
   defined, 69
   diagnosis competencies, 36
   education competencies, 55
   educational preparation for, 20–24
   environmental health competencies, 67–68
   ethics competencies, 53
   evaluation competencies, 50–51
   evidence-based practice and research competencies, 56
   health teaching and promotion competencies, 47
   implementation competencies, 43–44
   leadership competencies, 60–61

Advanced practice registered nurses
(*cont'd*)
  nursing process and, 6–8
  outcomes identification
    competencies, 38
  in outpatient settings, 6–8
  pain therapies and, 14
  planning competencies, 41
  prescriptive authority and treatment,
    2, 8, 14, 20, 29
    competencies, 49
  professional practice evaluation
    competencies, 64
  quality of practice competencies, 58
  resource utilization competencies, 62
  See also Graduate-level-prepared
    rheumatology nurses;
    Rheumatology registered nurses
Advocacy in rheumatology nursing
  practice, 11, 15, 28–29
  competencies involving, 42, 45, 47,
    52, 65, 67, 68
Age-appropriate care in rheumatology
  nursing practice, 15–20, 64
  See also Cultural competence and
    sensitivity
Alteration in comfort: stiffness
  Outcome Standard for Rheumatology
    Nursing Practice [1983], 82
Alteration in energy level: fatigue
  Outcome Standard for
    Rheumatology Nursing Practice
    [1983], 83
American College of Rheumatology
  (ACR), 22
American Nurses Association (ANA), 22, vi
  *Code of Ethics for Nurses with
    Interpretive Statements*, 25, 27, 28
  *Core Curriculum for Rheumatology
    Nurses*, 23
  Nursing: A Social Policy Statement, 81
  *Rheumatology Nursing: Scope and
    Standards of Practice*, 1, 2, 28
American Rheumatology Health
  Association (ARHA), 22
ANA. *See* American Nurses Association
  (ANA)

Analysis in rheumatology nursing
  practice. *See* Critical thinking,
  analysis, and synthesis
Anemia, rheumatic disease and, 5
Ankle arthritis, history, 3
Ankylosing spondylitis, 17, 18
  ASAS (disease activity index) for,
    50, 70
  genetics of, 26
APNCWG. *See* Advanced Practice
  Nursing Consensus Work Group
  (APNCWG)
APRNs. *See* Advanced practice registered
  nurses (APRNs)
ARHA. *See* American Rheumatology
  Health Association (ARHA)
ARHP. *See* Association of Rheumatology
  Health Professionals (ARHP)
Arthritis, 3–5, 81
  See also Rheumatoid arthritis (RA)
Arthritis Foundation, 22
ASAS (ankylosing spondylitis assessment
  score), 50, 70
  See also Ankylosing spondylitis
Aspirin, in arthritis, 3
Assessment in rheumatology nursing
  practice, 8
  APRN and, 6
  assessment data and its usage, 34, 35,
    36, 50
  competencies involving, 34–35
  disease activity indices for, 70
  health assessment questionnaire
    (HAQ), 70
  physical, 5
  Standard of Practice, 34–35
  techniques and tools for, 35, 50, 70
Association of Rheumatology Health
  Professionals (ARHP), 22
Autoimmune diseases
  rheumatology registered nurses
    and, 1
  definition, 70–71
  See also Rheumatic diseases

Autonomy in rheumatology nursing practice, 1, 52, 60

B

"Baby boomers," 16

Bayer Company, 3

Benefits and cost. *See* Cost and economic controls

Biologics (BRMs), 4, 5, 12
defined, 69

BRMs. *See* Biologics (BRMs)

Budgetary issues. *See* Cost and economic controls

Bullying, 25

C

Care and caring in rheumatology nursing practice
acute care settings (*See* Acute care settings)
caregivers of older adults, 18–19
child care and, 4, 20
coordination of care, 5–6, 19, 45
follow-up care, 7
self-care, 7
spiritual and emotional care, 34, 39, 46

Care delivery in rheumatology nursing practice, 45, 59
See also Coordination of care

Care recipients. *See* Healthcare consumers

Care standards. *See* Standards of Practice

Caregivers of older adults, 18–19

Centers for Medicare and Medicaid Services (CMS), 29

Certification and credentialing in rheumatology nursing practice, 22–23, 58

Children, rheumatology nurses and, 15–16, 19

Clients. *See* Healthcare consumers

Clinical trials, rheumatology registered nurses in, 10

Cloroquine, in arthritis, 4

CMS. *See* Centers for Medicare and Medicaid Services (CMS)

Code of Ethics for Nurses with Interpretive Statements (ANA), 25, 27, 28

Code of Federal Regulations (CFR), 11

Coding for payment and reimbursement (ICD-10-CM), 29

Collaboration in rheumatology nursing practice, 8, 14
competencies involving, 43, 50, 62–63
Standard of Professional Performance, 62–63
See also Communication; Interprofessional health care

Collegiality in rheumatology nursing practice. *See* Collaboration; Interprofessional health care; Peer review and relations

Communication in rheumatology nursing practice
competencies involving, 34, 43, 45, 46, 48, 59, 60, 62, 63, 67
Standards of Professional Performance, 59
See also Collaboration; Conflict resolution

Competencies for rheumatology nursing practice
for APRNs, 35, 36, 38, 41, 43–44, 45, 47, 48, 49, 50–51, 52–53, 55, 56, 58, 59, 60–61, 63, 64, 66, 67–68
assessment, 34–35
collaboration, 43, 50, 62–63
communication, 34, 43, 45, 46, 48, 59, 60, 62, 63, 67
consultation, 48
coordination of care, 45
defined, 69
diagnosis, 36
education, 54–55
environmental health, 67–68
ethics, 52–53

Competencies for rheumatology nursing
practice (*cont'd*)
evaluation, 50–51
evidence-based practice and research,
56
for graduate-level-prepared
rheumatology nurses
(*See* Graduate-level-prepared
rheumatology nurses)
health teaching and promotion,
46–47
implementation, 42–44
leadership, 60–61
outcomes identification, 37–38
planning, 39–41
prescriptive authority and treatment, 49
professional practice evaluation, 64
quality of practice, 57–58
resource utilization, 65–66
See also Advanced practice
registered nurses (APRNs);
Cultural competence and
sensitivity; Graduate-level-
prepared rheumatology nurses;
Rheumatology registered nurses;
Standards of Practice; Standards
of Professional Performance

Complementary/alternative therapies,
defined, 43, 69

Confidentiality and privacy in
rheumatology nursing practice, 10,
15, 28
competencies involving, 35, 52
See also Ethics

Conflict resolution, 59, 60

Consensus Model for APRN
Regulation, 21, 23

Consultation in rheumatology nursing
practice, 8, 12
competencies involving, 48
Standard of Practice, 48

Continuing education in rheumatology
nursing practice, 22

Contraceptive counseling, 17

Coordination of care in rheumatology
nursing practice, 5–6, 19

competencies involving, 45
Standard of Practice, 45

*Core Curriculum for Rheumatology
Nurses* (ANA), 23

Cost and economic controls in
rheumatology nursing practice, 5,
19, 25
competencies involving, 37, 38, 49, 57,
65, 66
coverage and reimbursement issues,
11

Counseling in rheumatology nursing
practice, 11, 16, 17

Coverage, laws, regulations, and policies
and, 11

Credentialing in rheumatology nursing
practice. *See* Certification and
credentialing

Criteria in Outcome Standards for
Rheumatology Nursing Practice
[1983]
alteration in comfort: stiffness, 82
alteration in energy level: fatigue, 83
disturbance in self-concept, 88
ineffective coping, individual or
family, 87
knowledge deficit regarding physical
mobility (ambulation), 85
knowledge deficit regarding self-
management decisions, 86
self-care deficit, 84

Critical thinking, analysis, and synthesis
in rheumatology nursing practice, 4,
12, 35, 41, 45, 47, 48, 55, 58
See also Evidence-based practice
and research; Knowledge, skills,
abilities, and judgment; Nursing
process

Cultural competence and sensitivity in
rheumatology nursing practice
assessment and, 34
competencies involving, 34, 37, 39,
42, 46, 47, 64
health teaching and promotion and,
46, 47
implementation and, 42

outcomes identification and, 37
planning and, 39
professional practice evaluation and, 64

Cultural factors, for rheumatic condition, 17–18

Curriculum content in rheumatology nursing practice, 23

D

DAS-28 (Disease Activity Score 28), 50, 70

Data and information in rheumatology nursing practice
assessment data usage, 34, 35, 36, 50
competencies involving, 34, 35, 36, 41, 42, 45, 48, 50, 57
See also Assessment; Diagnosis

Decision-making in rheumatology nursing practice
competencies involving, 36, 48, 52, 53, 59, 60, 62, 64, 65

Delegation in rheumatology nursing practice, 65

Dementia, 16, 19

Depression in rheumatology nursing patients, 15, 18

Diagnosis in rheumatology nursing practice
APRN and, 6
assessment data and, 34
competencies involving, 34, 35, 36, 41, 42, 49, 50
defined, 69
diagnostic tests and processes, 6, 7, 35, 36, 41, 49
rheumatology registered nurses and, 2
Standard of Practice, 36

Dietary issues and rheumatology nursing patients, 18, 27
See also Nutritional issues

Dignity in rheumatology nursing practice, 26, 45, 52, 60
See also Ethics

Disability in rheumatology nursing practice, 11, 20

Disease activity indices, defined, 70

Disease-modifying antirheumatic drugs (DMARDs), 1, 4, 5, 12
defined, 70

Disturbance in self-concept
Outcome Standard for Rheumatology Nursing Practice [1983], 88

DMARDs. *See* Disease-modifying antirheumatic drugs (DMARDs)

Doctorate in Nursing Practice (DNP), 22

Documentation in rheumatology nursing practice, 11
assessment and, 35
collaboration and, 62, 63
competencies involving, 35, 36, 37, 40, 43, 45, 50, 56, 57, 62, 63
coordination of care and, 45
diagnosis and, 36
EHR and, 14–15
evaluation and, 50
evidence-based practice and research and, 56
implementation and, 43
outcomes identification and, 37
planning and, 40
quality of practice and, 57

Driving, rheumatic disease and, 4

E

Economic controls in rheumatology nursing practice. *See* Cost and economic controls

Education in rheumatology nursing practice
competencies involving, 49, 54–55, 56, 60, 63
curriculum content, 23
educational preparation for rheumatology nursing, 20–24
of healthcare consumer, 1, 5, 7, 10–11, 14, 18–19

Education in rheumatology nursing practice (*cont'd*)
in pediatric nursing, 15
Rheumatology Nursing: Scope and Standards of Practice in, 2
Standard of Professional Performance, 54–55

Egyptian mummies, arthritis, 3

EHRs. *See* Electronic health records (EHRs)

Elderly populations, 18–19
See also Population-based health care

Electronic health records (EHRs) in rheumatology nursing, 14–15, 42

Emotional and psychosocial issues of patients, 4, 5, 6, 12, 13, 14, 30, 34

Environmental factors, for rheumatic conditions, 17–18

Environmental health and safety in rheumatology nursing practice, 17, 26, 27
competencies involving, 34, 36, 39, 46–47, 54, 58, 67–68
Standard of Professional Performance, 67–68

Environments for rheumatology nursing practice, 5–11, 17
acute care settings (*See* Acute care settings)
infusion suites, 5–8
other settings, 9–10
outpatient settings, 5–8
research facilities, 10–11
workplace safety, 25

Errors, medical, 59

Ethical decision-making in rheumatology nursing practice, 35

Ethics in rheumatology nursing practice, 27–28
competencies involving, 52–53, 57
ethical decision-making, 35
Standard of Professional Performance, 52–53
workplace safety, 25

Evaluation in rheumatology nursing practice
competencies involving, 50–51
Standards of Practice, 50–51
See also Expected outcomes; Professional practice evaluation

Evidence-based practice and research in rheumatology nursing practice, 11–12
competencies involving, 56
defined, 70
Standard of Professional Performance, 56

Expected outcomes in rheumatology nursing practice, 9
attainment of, 50
diagnosis and, 36
evaluation and, 50
outcomes identification and, 37
planning and, 39
See also Evaluation; Outcomes identification; Planning

F

Families and rheumatology nursing practice
assessment, 34, 35
collaboration and, 62, 63
communication and, 59
coordination of care and, 45
defined, 70
diagnosis and, 36
environmental health and, 67
ethics and, 52
evaluation and, 50
health teaching and promotion and, 46, 47
as healthcare consumers, 65
implementation and, 42, 43
leadership and, 61
outcomes identification and, 37
planning and, 39, 40
rheumatology registered nurses
and diagnosis of disease, 2
education, 1, 5, 14, 15, 18–19
psychosocial support, 6

RNS commitment, 1
See also Healthcare consumers

Family and Medical Leave Act, 11

Fatigue, Outcome Standard for Rheumatology Nursing Practice [1983], 83

Financial issues in rheumatology nursing practice, 5
See also Cost and economic controls
Fibromyalgia, 18

Follows up in rheumatology nursing practice, 7

Food and Drug Administration (FDA), 17

Franklin, Benjamin, 4

The Future of Nursing: Leading Change, Advancing Health, 21

G

Genetics and genomics in rheumatology nursing practice, 17, 26–27

Geriatric population, rheumatology nurses and, 18–19, 20
See also Population-based health care

Gold salt treatments, in arthritis, 4

Gout, 3, 4, 18
See also Arthritis

Graduate-level-prepared rheumatology nurses, 14
assessment competencies, 35
collaboration competencies, 63
communication competencies, 59
consultation competencies, 48
coordination of care competencies, 45
diagnosis competencies, 36
education competencies, 55
environmental health competencies, 67–68
ethics competencies, 53
evaluation competencies, 50–51
evidence-based practice and research competencies, 56

health teaching and promotion competencies, 47
implementation competencies, 43–44
leadership competencies, 60–61
outcomes identification competencies, 38
planning competencies, 41
professional practice evaluation competencies, 64
quality of practice competencies, 58
resource utilization competencies, 66

Graduate-level-prepared specialty nurse, defined, 70

H

Health assessment questionnaire (HAQ), 70

Health teaching and promotion in rheumatology nursing practice, 43, 67
competencies involving, 46–47
Standard of Practice, 46–47
See also Promotive rheumatology nursing practice

Healthcare consumers, 65
challenges in activities, 4–5
coverage and reimbursement issues, 11
defined, 70
diagnosis of disease, 2
education, 1, 5, 7, 10–11, 14, 18–19
follows up, 7
in infusion suite, 8–9
interprofessional teams, 24–25
nursing process for, APRN and, 6–8
in outpatient settings, 5–11
psychosocial support, 6
responsibility of, 1
Rheumatology Nursing: Scope and Standards of Practice for, 2
rheumatology registered nurses and, 1–2, 5–6
RNS commitment, 1
in self-care, 7
See also Families; Population-based health care

Healthcare providers in rheumatology nursing practice, 4
defined, 70

Healthcare setting, 1, 5–11

Healthy lifestyle issues in rheumatology nursing patients, 9, 27, 46
See also Dietary issues; Nutritional issues; Smoking; Weight management issues

Heart disease, rheumatic disease and, 5

HLA-B27 gene, 17, 26–27

Hoffman, Felix, 3

Hypertension, rheumatoid arthritis and, 18

I

ICD-10-CM. See International Statistical Classification of Diseases and Related Health Problems, 10th Revision, Clinical Modification

Immune-mediated diseases, defined, 70–71

Implementation in rheumatology nursing practice, 6–7, 11
competencies involving, 42–44
pain management plan, 14
Standard of Practice, 42–44

Ineffective coping, individual or family Outcome Standard for Rheumatology Nursing Practice [1983], 87

Infection in rheumatic disease, 12, 18

Information in rheumatology nursing practice, 9, 10, 12, 14–15, 30–31
See also Data and information

Infusible medications in rheumatic conditions, 9
side-effects, 9

Infusion suites in rheumatology nursing practice, 8–9

Institute for Medicine (IOM), 21, 22

Interdisciplinary health care in rheumatology nursing practice. See Interprofessional health care

International Conference on Harmonization (ICH), 11

International Statistical Classification of Diseases and Related Health Problems, 10th Revision, Clinical Modification (ICD-10-CM), 29

Interprofessional competencies in rheumatology nursing practice, 41, 45, 53, 57, 59, 60, 61, 63, 66
See also Collaboration

Interprofessional health care in rheumatology nursing practice, 45
See also Coordination of care

Interprofessional teams
RN and healthcare consumer, 24–25

Interprofessionalism, defined, 71

Interventions in rheumatology nursing practice, 6, 38, 41, 42, 50, 81

Investigator, defined, 71

IOM. See Institute for Medicine (IOM)

J

Judgment in rheumatology nursing practice, 4, 54, 55, 61
See also Knowledge, skills, abilities, and judgment

K

Knowledge, skills, abilities, and judgment in rheumatology nursing practice, 1, 4, 11
assessment competencies, 34, 35
collaboration and, 62
competencies involving, 34, 35, 41, 42, 43, 49, 54, 55, 56, 61, 62, 67
education competencies, 54, 55
environmental health and, 67
evidence-based practice and research competencies, 56
implementation competencies, 42, 43
leadership competencies, 61
planning competencies, 41

prescriptive authority and treatment competencies, 49
See also Critical thinking, analysis, and synthesis; Education; Evidence-based practice and research

Knowledge deficit regarding physical mobility (ambulation)
Outcome Standard for Rheumatology Nursing Practice [1983], 85

Knowledge deficit regarding self-management decisions
Outcome Standard for Rheumatology Nursing Practice [1983], 86

L

Laws, statutes, and regulations in rheumatology nursing practice, 21, 25, 29
APRNs, 8, 10, 14, 20, 21
competencies involving, 35, 40, 50, 52, 65
coverage and reimbursement and, 11
prescriptive authority and treatment, 49
professional practice and regulation, 64
See also Consensus Model for APRN Regulation

Leadership in rheumatology nursing practice
competencies involving, 45, 58, 60–61
Standard of Professional Performance, 60–61

Learning in rheumatology nursing practice, 14, 21
See also Education

Legal issues. *See* Laws, statutes, and regulations

Licensing and licensure in rheumatology nursing practice, 21, 23

Licensure, Accreditation, Certification and Education (LACE), 21, 23

Life-threatening infusion reactions, 8

Low-income assistance programs, 5

Lung disease, rheumatic disease and, 5

Lupus. *See* Systemic lupus erythematosus

M

Medical errors, 59

Medicare Part B and D options, 5

Medications in rheumatology nursing practice, 1, 3–5, 30
advocacy and, 28
age-specific, 15, 17, 19
biologics (BRMs), 4, 5, 12
competencies involving,
DMARDs, 1, 4, 5, 12, 70
EHRs and, 14, 15
infusible, 8–9
interactions, 5, 14
pain management, 13, 14
polypharmacy, 14
population-specific, 15, 17, 19
rehabilitation, 27
research, 10, 11
steroids, 4, 12
See also Prescriptive authority

Mummies, arthritis in, 3

N

National Council of State Boards of Nursing APRN Advisory Committee (NCSBN), 21, 23

NCSBN. *See* National Council of State Boards of Nursing APRN Advisory Committee (NCSBN)

Nonsteroidal antiinflammatory drugs (NSAIDs), 1

North Americans, 3

Nursesbooks.org, vi

Nursing, 81
defined, 71

Nursing: A Social Policy Statement (ANA), 81

Nursing activities. *See* Activities

Nursing care. *See* Care and caring

Nursing care activities, 11

Nursing competence. *See* Competencies

Nursing education. *See* Education

Nursing interventions. *See* Interventions

Nursing judgment. *See* Knowledge, skills, abilities, and judgment

Nursing plan, for acute and chronic pain issues, 13

Nursing practice, defined, 71

Nursing process, 33
  APRN and, 6–8
  defined, 71
  pain management and, 13
  See also Standards of Practice; Specific standards

Nursing specialty, core curriculum in, 23

Nursing standards. *See* Standards of Practice; Standards of Professional Performance

Nutrition and rheumatology nursing patients, 9, 13, 16, 19, 46, 69

O

Obesity, rheumatoid arthritis and, 18

Older adults, rheumatology nurses and, 18–19
  See also Population-based health care

Osteoarthritis, history, 3

Osteoporosis, 3, 16

Outcome Standard for Rheumatology Nursing Practice [1983], 81–88
  alteration in comfort: stiffness, 82
  alteration in energy level: fatigue, 83
  disturbance in self-concept, 88
  ineffective coping, individual or family, 87
  knowledge deficit regarding physical mobility (ambulation), 85

knowledge deficit regarding self-management decisions, 86
  self-care deficit, 84

Outcomes identification in rheumatology nursing practice, 6
  competencies involving, 37–38
  Standard of Practice, 37–38
  See also Planning

Outpatient settings in rheumatology nursing practice, 5–8, 21–22

P

Pain management in rheumatology nursing practice, 12–14

Patient. *See* Healthcare consumer

Pediatric population, rheumatology nurses and, 15–16, 19
  See also Population-based health care

Peer review and relations in rheumatology nursing practice, 16, 20, 22, 25
  collaboration and, 62
  competencies involving, 54, 56, 62, 64
  education and, 54
  evidence-based practice and research and, 56
  professional practice evaluation and, 64
  See also Collaboration; Communication

Pharma-sponsored copay assistance, 5

Physical assessments in rheumatology nursing practice, 5

Planning in rheumatology nursing practice
  competencies involving, 39–41
  consultation and, 48
  diagnostic plans, 8
  evaluation and, 50, 51
  implementation of plan, 42–44
  outcomes identification and, 37
  resources utilization and, 65

Standard of Practice, 39–41
treatment and therapeutic plans, 2, 6, 13, 18, 19

Policies in rheumatology nursing practice
competencies involving, 35, 51, 57, 60, 65, 67
developing, 2
procedures and, 2

Polymyalgia rheumatica, 16

Polypharmacy, 14

Population-based health care
rheumatology nurses and, 15–20
adult, 16–18, 20
geriatric, 18–19, 20
pediatric, 15–16, 19

Practice environments and settings in rheumatology nursing practice, 5–11
acute care settings (*See* Acute care settings)
infusion suites, 8–9
other settings, 9–10
outpatient settings, 5–8
research facilities, 10–11

Pregnancy, rheumatic diseases in, 4, 16–17

Prescriptive authority and treatment in rheumatology nursing practice, 1, 2, 7, 8, 9
APRNs, 2, 8, 14, 20, 29
competencies involving, 49
Standard of Practice, 49

Preventive practice in healthcare and rheumatology nursing practice
competencies involving, 39, 46, 47

Privacy in rheumatology nursing practice. *See* Confidentiality and privacy

Procedures in rheumatology nursing practice, 8

Professional development and rheumatology nursing practice
competencies involving, 64

Professional practice evaluation in rheumatology nursing practice

competencies involving, 64
Standard of Professional Performance, 64

Promotive rheumatology nursing practice, 7
competencies involving, 43, 46, 47, 56, 59, 61, 62, 65, 67
health teaching and promotion and, 46–47

Psoriatic arthritis, 3

Psychosocial and emotional issues of patients, 4, 5, 6, 12, 13, 14, 30, 34

Q

Quality of practice in rheumatology nursing practice
competencies involving, 57–58
Standard of Professional Performance, 57–58

Quinine, in arthritis, 4

R

Registered nurse (RN), defined, 71

Regulatory and statutory issues in rheumatology nursing practice. *See* Laws, statutes, and regulations

Rehabilitation in rheumatology nursing practice, 27

Reimbursement, laws, regulations, and policies and, 11

Renoir, Auguste, 4

Repetitive movements, rheumatoid arthritis and, 18

Reproductive health concerns
children with rheumatic condition and, 16

Research in rheumatology nursing practice
competencies involving, 40, 41, 47, 54, 55, 56, 58, 63
facilities, rheumatology registered nurses in, 10–11

Resource utilization in rheumatology nursing practice
competencies involving, 65–66
Standard of Professional Performance, 65–66

Responsibility in rheumatology nursing practice, 1
competencies involving, 43, 48, 50, 57, 65
of healthcare consumer, 1
of rheumatology registered nurses, 11–12
assessment techniques and tools, 50, 70
defined, 71
disease activity indices, 70
genetics of, 26–27
See also Rheumatoid arthritis; Systemic lupus erythematosus

Rheumatic diseases, 3–5, 16, 18

Rheumatoid arthritis (RA), 1, 3–5, 16–17, 18, 34, 36, 39, 41, 42

Rheumatology, defined, 3

Rheumatology Nurses Society (RNS), 1, 22, vi

Rheumatology nursing, defined, 3

Rheumatology nursing practice
EHRs in, 14–15
environments, 5–11
acute care settings (See Acute care settings)
infusion suites, 8–9
other settings, 9–10
outpatient settings, 5–8
research facilities, 10–11
family history, 17
Outcome Standards [1983], 81–88 (See also Outcome Standard for Rheumatology Nursing Practice [1983])
pain management in, 12–14
scope (See Scope of Rheumatology Nursing Practice)
standards (See Standards of Rheumatology Nursing Practice)
trends and issues in, 25–29
advocacy, 28–29
ethics, 27–28
genetic factors, 26–27
ICD-10-CM, 29
rehabilitation, 27
workplace safety, 26

Rheumatology registered nurses, 1, 4
accountability, 2
action regarding adverse events, 2
in acute care settings (See Acute care settings)
administration of infusible medications, 1–2
advocacy, 28–29
assessment competencies, 34–35
autoimmune and inflammatory diseases, 1
in clinical trials, 10
collaboration competencies, 62
communication competencies, 59
coordination of care competencies, 45
coverage and reimbursement issues, 11
diagnosis competencies, 36
diagnosis of disease and, 2
education competencies, 54
educational preparation for, 20–24
EHRs use and, 14–15
environmental health competencies, 67–68
ethics competencies, 52
evaluation competencies, 50
evidence-based practice and research competencies, 56
in faith community, 10
health teaching and promotion competencies, 46–47
healthcare consumer, education, 1, 5, 10–11, 14
implementation competencies, 42–43
in infusion suites, 8–9
interprofessional teams, 24–25
leadership competencies, 60
other settings, 9–10
outcomes identification competencies, 37
in outpatient settings, 5–6

pain management and (*See* Pain management)

planning competencies, 39–40

populations served by (*See* Population-based health care, rheumatology nurses and)

professional practice evaluation competencies, 64

quality of practice competencies, 57–58

in research facilities, 10–11

resource utilization competencies, 65

roles and responsibilities, 11–12

in schools, 10

Risks and risk management in rheumatology nursing practice, 5

competencies involving, 36, 37, 46, 47, 53, 59, 65, 67

RNS. *See* Rheumatology Nurses Society (RNS)

Roles, of rheumatology registered nurses, 11–12

S

Safety in rheumatology nursing practice, 19

competencies involving, 36, 40, 42, 43, 46, 52, 57, 63, 65, 67

workplace safety, 25

See also Environmental health and safety

Salicin, (acetylsalicylic acid), 3 for pain, 3

Scope of Rheumatology Nursing Practice, 3–31

defined, 71

EHRs in, 14–15

environments, 5–11

acute care settings (*See* Acute care settings)

infusion suites, 8–9

other settings, 9–10

outpatient settings, 5–8

research facilities, 10–11

history, 3–5

pain management, 12–14

population-based health care (*See* Population-based health care)

roles and responsibilities of rheumatology nurses, 11–12

summary, 29–31

trends and issues in, 25–29

advocacy, 28–29

ethics, 27–28

genetic factors, 26–27

ICD-10-CM, 29

rehabilitation, 27

workplace safety, 26

Self-administered and self-injected medications, 13, 43

Self-care, and rheumatology nursing patients, 7, 13, 46

deficit, Outcome Standard for Rheumatology Nursing Practice [1983], 84

See also Healthy lifestyle

Self-esteem and self-esteem rheumatology nursing patients, 15, 19, 20

Settings for rheumatology nursing practice. *See* Practice environments and settings

Sexual activity, rheumatic disease and, 4

Side-effects profiles and monitoring, 1, 5, 8, 9

SLEDAI (systemic lupus erythematosus disease activity index), 70

See also Systemic lupus erythematosus

Smoking, 5, 17–18

Specialty of rheumatology nursing, 1, 20, 22

organizations, 22

Rheumatology Nursing: Scope and Standards of Practice in, 2

Spiritual care in rheumatology nursing practice, 34

competencies involving, 39, 46

Spondylarthropathies, 3

Standardized language and classification systems in rheumatology nursing practice, 36, 40

Standards, defined, 72

Standards of Practice for Rheumatology Nursing, 34–51
assessment, 34–35
consultation, 48
coordination of care, 45
diagnosis, 36
evaluation, 50–51
health teaching and promotion, 46–47
implementation, 42–44
outcomes identification, 37–38
planning, 39–41
prescriptive authority and treatment, 49
See also Standards of Professional Performance; Specific standards

Standards of Professional Performance for Rheumatology Nursing, 52–68
collaboration, 62–63
communication, 59
defined, 72
education, 54–55
environmental health, 67–68
ethics, 52–53
evidence-based practice and research, 56
leadership, 60–61
professional practice evaluation, 64
quality of practice, 57–58
resource utilization, 65–66
See also Specific standards

Standards of Rheumatology Nursing Practice, 2, 33–68
See also Standards of Practice; Standards of Professional Performance

Statutes in rheumatology nursing practice. See Laws, statutes, and regulations

Steroids, in arthritis, 4, 12

Stiffness, Outcome Standard for Rheumatology Nursing Practice [1983], 82

Subinvestigator, defined, 72

Synthesis in rheumatology nursing practice, 4, 12, 35, 41, 45, 47, 48, 55, 58

Systemic lupus erythematosus (SLE), 1, 3, 18, 34, 35, 36, 42
disease activity index for, 70
genetics of, 26

T

Technological-based competencies in rheumatology nursing practice, 39, 42, 46, 63, 65

Treatment and therapeutic plans in rheumatology nursing practice, 2, 6, 13, 18, 19
See also Planning

Treatment and therapy prescription in rheumatology nursing practice, 2, 6, 7, 14
See also Prescriptive authority and treatment

V

Values, attitudes, and beliefs in rheumatology nursing practice, 34, 37, 39, 41, 46, 47, 52
See also Cultural competence and sensitivity

Vasculitis, 1, 3

Violence, workplace, 25

W

Weight management issues in rheumatology nursing practice, 27, 39, 46

WHO. See World Health Organization (WHO)

Willow bark, for pain, 3

Women in rheumatology nursing practice, 16, 17, 18

See also Population-based
  health care

Work and practice environments for
  rheumatology nursing practice
  assessment and, 34
  collaboration and, 62
  communication and, 59
  competencies involving, 34, 39, 46,
    54, 58, 59, 60, 62, 67–68
  education and, 54
  environmental health and, 67–68

health teaching and promotion
  and, 46
leadership and, 60
planning and, 39
quality of practice and, 58
workplace safety, 25
See also Health teaching and
  promotion

Workplace issues. *See* Work and practice
  environments

World Health Organization (WHO), 29